Cancer: through the eyes of ten women

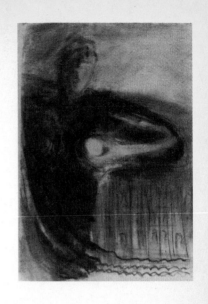

The Egg

Cancer:
through the eyes of ten women

Edited by Patricia Duncker and Vicky Wilson

Drawings by Catherine Arthur

An Imprint of HarperCollins*Publishers*

To Catherine Arthur,
Linda Brandon and Sue Goddard

Pandora
An Imprint of HarperCollins*Publishers*
77–85 Fulham Palace Road,
Hammersmith, London W6 8JB

1160 Battery Street,
San Francisco, California 94111–1213
Published by Pandora 1996
1   3   5   7   9   10   8   6   4   2

The contributors assert the moral right to
be identified as the authors of this work

A catalogue record for this book
is available from the British Library

ISBN 0 04 440980 X

Printed in Great Britain by
Caledonian International Book Manufacturing Ltd, Glasgow

Contents

Acknowledgements

The translation from the French of Jacqueline Julien's 'Sweat' is by Armelle Tardiveau and Vicky Wilson. The photography of Catherine Arthur's drawings is by Julie Millard.

Marilyn Hacker's poems have appeared in *Winter Numbers: Poems* (W. W. Norton, 1994). Hilda Raz's 'For Barbara, Who Brings Me a Green Stone in the Shape of a Triangle' has appeared in *The Bread Loaf Anthology of Contemporary Nature Poetry* and *The Women's Review of Books*; 'Bernini's Ribbon' in *Nebraska English Journal*; 'Weathering/Boundaries/What Is Good' in *Literature and Medicine*; 'Breast/Fever' in *Ploughshares*; and 'Petting the Scar' in *The Southern Review*. Jackie Stacey's 'Conquering Heroes: The Politics of Cancer Narratives' is a revised version of the opening chapter of her book-length study of these issues, *Teratologies – A Cultural Study of Cancer* (Routledge, 1997).

Our thanks to Belinda Budge for her continuing faith in this project.

List of Contributors

Catherine Rae Arthur (1937–91) emigrated from England to Canada in 1963. Always a seeker, she threw herself into painting, poetry and some tumultuous relationships. She worked as a technical journalist, becoming Features Editor of *Printing World*. Aged 48, she gave up her job to study art, graduating in 1989. Twelve months later breast cancer (with spread in the spine) was diagnosed. She produced the 'Cancer Drawings: Another Way of Seeing' when already seriously ill. Her work has been exhibited in London at the Whitechapel, Lauderdale House, the LLGC and Centerprise, and written about in *Feminist Review*.

Carole Colbourn spent her earliest years on the largest council estate in the UK. Having been accepted to do French at university she decided that she really wanted to be a doctor after a chance encounter with a medical student, and after watching *Gone with the Wind*. Two years into the course at Newcastle she met an agric, Phil, who promptly moved to London to do a Ph.D. at Imperial College. Carole transferred to the Middlesex Hospital Medical School. During her course, she spent time working at Mission hospitals in Nigeria. They married in 1972 and have since lived in six homes, with increasingly large gardens, in various parts of the country. They have three children. In the course of their life they have been Anglicans, Baptists, various shades of Charismatic and Evangelical, and are now card-carrying Methodists. Carole had her mastectomy in 1989.

Evelyn Alexandra Dale was born in 1968 in Hitchin, Hertfordshire. In 1988, she read Classics at St Hilda's College, Oxford, and graduated in 1992. In 1989, at the age of 20, she was diagnosed as suffering from breast cancer and was believed to be the youngest patient nationally to be treated for this type of cancer. In 1994, after qualifying as a teacher, she underwent further surgery for breast cancer. She is currently studying journalism at the London College of Printing. She has had several articles published in the *Evening Standard*. She now lives in London.

Debbie Dickinson has worked in the music business, primarily with jazz-related musicians, in management, production, and as a sound engineer and tour manager, for the best part of 20 years. She presently coordinates a major International Jazz Festival as well as touring internationally. She was diagnosed with bladder cancer at the age of 30 – eight years ago.

Patricia Duncker was born in the West Indies. She spent five years lecturing in France, where she still lives for part of the year. She now teaches writing and nineteenth-century literature at the University of Wales, Aberystwyth. She is the author of *Sisters and Strangers: An Introduction to Contemporary Feminist Fiction* (Blackwell, 1992) and *Hallucinating Foucault* (Serpent's Tail, 1996). She had ardenocarcinoma, a rare, aggressive form of cervical cancer, in 1986.

Dale Gunthorp was Catherine Arthur's partner from 1980 until the end of 1991. She is the author of *The Commonwealth Yearbook* (Hanson Cooke for the Commonwealth Secretariat, 1996–7), and, writing as Claire Macquet, of *Looking for Ammu* (Virago, 1992) and *The Flying Hart* (Sheba, 1991).

Marilyn Hacker lives in Paris and in Manhattan, with her life partner, AIDS practitioner Karyn London. She is the author of eight books, including the verse novel *Love, Death and the Changing of the Seasons*, which was published in the UK by Onlywomen Press, as was *The Hang-Glider's Daughter*, a selection of work from three of her American collections. Her most recent book, *Winter Numbers* (W.W. Norton, 1994) received a Lambda Literary Award and the Lenore Marshall Poetry Prize. The sequence 'Cancer Winter' was written during the winter and spring of 1993, while she was undergoing chemotherapy and working as editor of the *Kenyon Review*.

Jacqueline Julien was born in Morocco in 1945. She lived for many years in Italy, where she discovered the Women's Liberation Movement, and in Poland, where her son was born in 1974. For the last 20 years she has worked in publishing in Toulouse, France. She is committed to the dissemination of lesbian culture and is co-founder and president of the lesbian meeting place Bagdam Café, and executive editor of the monthly *Lesbia Magazine*. She is author of the self-published text and cassette *Le Feu, Chronique du désir*. She began to write 'Sweat' two months before learning she had breast cancer in 1994, and finished it two months after her mastectomy. Loved, desired and supported by the woman with whom she shares her life, she sees her cancer as a unique opportunity for physical, emotional, mental and spiritual clarification.

Hilda Raz is the author of two books of poems, *What Is Good* and *The Bone Dish*. Her poems, essays and reviews have appeared in magazines, anthologies and collections from Scribner's, Johns Hopkins University Press, University Press of New England, Longstreet Press, Bench Press and many others. Recent work appears or is forthcoming in *The Women's Review of Books*, *Ploughshares*, *The Southern Review*, *The Colorado Review* and *Literature and Medicine*. The poems given here are from *Divine Honors*, a manuscript collection, and her work on her experience with breast cancer includes 'Junk', an essay to be reprinted in *Worlds in Our Words: Contemporary American Women Writers*

(Prentice Hall, 1996). She is a professor of English at the University of Nebraska and the editor of *Prairie Schooner*, a venerable literary quarterly entering its seventieth year of continuous publication.

Cathy Read is a British doctor of medicine who works full-time as an author and journalist. Her main interests are health, medicine and the environment. She has written extensively in the medical and science press and for national newspapers and magazines in the UK. Her work has appeared in *The Guardian, The Independent, The Independent on Sunday, The Evening Standard, The Ecologist* and *Everywoman*. She is the author of *Preventing Breast Cancer: The Politics of an Epidemic* (HarperCollins, 1995). Cathy Read is currently based in Sheffield. She is married to a physician and has three children.

Felly Nkweto Simmonds was born in Zambia. She is a writer and lecturer in Sociology at the University of Northumbria, Newcastle upon Tyne. She had a mastectomy in February 1992 and has written on the experience of breast cancer, as a Black woman, in *The Guardian* ('Black and Blue About Pink', 4.11.93); *General Practitioner* ('Black Women Get Breast Cancer', 5.2.93); and *The Weekly Journal* ('You Have Breast Cancer', 12.8.93). She has a daughter and two sons, who continue to sustain her in her life as a new woman.

Jackie Stacey is a lecturer in the Sociology Department at Lancaster University, where she teaches Film Studies, Cultural Studies and Women's Studies. Her previous publications in these areas include *Off Centre: Feminism and Cultural Studies* (edited with Sarah Franklin and Celia Lury; Routledge, 1991); *Working Out: New Directions for Women's Studies* (edited with Ann Phoenix and Hilary Hinds; Falmer Press, 1992); *Star Gazing: Hollywood Cinema and Female Spectatorship* (Routledge, 1994); *Romance Revisited* (edited with Lynne Pearce; Lawrence and Wishart, 1995). In 1991 she was diagnosed with cancer following surgery and was treated with chemotherapy as well as with a number of alternative therapies, over the next six months. Since this time she has been writing personal/critical accounts of the changing health cultures that frame experiences of having cancer in contemporary society. The chapter in this collection is her first publication in this area and precedes the appearance of her book-length study of the subject entitled *Teratologies – A Cultural Study of Cancer* (Routledge, 1997).

Vicky Wilson has worked as an editor in publishing for 20 years in the areas of architecture, design, film and feminism. She was a co-founder of feminist publishers Scarlet Press in 1992. She lives in London with her one-year-old daughter.

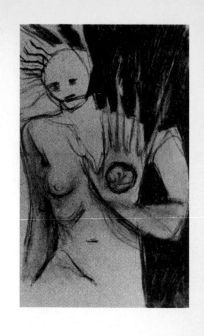

The Gestation

Preface

Writing, writing the truth, nothing is more difficult.
Jacqueline Julien

In this book you will find many metaphors for cancer. The disease is variously represented and described as the host, the guest, the mother, the child, the egg, the secret lover, the murderer, the terrorist, the addiction. All these metaphors are an attempt to tell a truth that can never be told directly; the truth about the experience of cancer. We first began work on *Cancer: through the eyes of ten women* in the autumn of 1991. Catherine Arthur, whose drawing sequence 'Another Way of Seeing' structures the book, was dying. She died on 1 December that year. Her sequence is a method of interpreting her cancer, re-interpreting her body and constructing her own cancer narrative – literally, 'another way of seeing'.

This book has taken five years to complete. The women to whom it is dedicated had either wanted to contribute or left us their work when they died.

One of the characteristics of cancer is its intimacy. It is a disease that you produce in your own body. Hence the intimacy of the relationships indicated by the metaphors we have used: mother, lover, murderer. Cancer usually takes a long time to kill you. Thus you have time to search through layers of memories, to know your own dying. Even when you are pronounced 'cured' you are forced to return for tests, check-ups, scans, probes, biopsies, year after year. You can never escape the fact that you have had cancer. The ghost of the disease, or the disease itself, remains with you.

Many of the writers here indicate the ambiguity of their experience, the way in which what happened shifts, changes, metamorphoses in memory and on the page. The drama of hospitals, diagnoses and treatments are easier to describe than the long, spectral relationship with the past, the others around us, memory and the self. The disease changes us, but it is in itself changed; by the work of understanding, remembering, forgetting. Most of us who survive the disease have to live in new bodies, or bodies that are new to us. We may now mistrust this unknown body, or the old body which has betrayed us. We may no longer love ourselves, we may no longer be loveable, we may no longer be loved.

Cancer appears to be generated from within the body. We are only beginning to identify the sources of cancer: environmental, genetic, possibly viral or influenced by diet. It has therefore always been tempting to see the woman who has cancer as responsible for her own disease. You can reject this, enraged, as I did, or play with the idea that your cancer belongs to you: that you have made it yourself and can therefore unmake it again. This is a way of regaining control over your own life, your own illness and your own death.

When we decided to create this book I asked for writing that did not reproduce what I began to realise was 'The Cancer Narrative'. This is what I wrote:

I am asking several other women who either have or have had cancer to write an essay or a contribution in another form, to interrogate what this illness has given to you or taken away from your life. I would like you to ask yourselves how the fact of cancer has affected your relationships, your work, your family, your sexuality and the meaning you give to your own body. How has cancer changed the way in which you live your life and the terms within which you understand your own death? There is very little sensible or sensitive writing about death that does not slide either into a morass of sentimentality or nihilistic metaphysics. I would like to feel that we could confront our own deaths with both fear and courage. But above all I would like to make a clear space where we can use our own experience to think, to reflect, to meditate, to make art.

I am not looking for heartening tales of noble survival, either, if that wasn't how it was. Cancer is terrifying, debilitating, depressing and potentially murderous. It need not be illuminating nor revealing in existential ways. The legacy can be bitterness, waste, loss and the perpetual fear of becoming ill again. If that has been the case, say so. In my own reading about cancer, attempting to come to terms with my own illness, I found myself perpetually reading what I now call 'the cancer narrative'. This is the ennobling tale of caring solidarity where love conquers death. The narrative may end in death, never gruesome or painful, or in survival, but it is always, finally, a Great Triumph of the Human Spirit. No doubt these tales are a lot easier to publish than anything harder to hear and more rigorous to read. But I read them with slowly accumulating fury. Nowhere did I read what I had lived through. I am not casting doubt on the authenticity of survival stories. So far, eight years on, I too have survived. But I would like to feel that we can confront the metaphysical darkness, which may be what we have seen, head on.

I envisage an abstract, essentially philosophical book – a thinking about cancer. No woman who has had cancer continues her life unchanged. I would like you to focus on that change, the shape that change has taken in your life and your work, your thinking about others and the meanings you found in your life, whatever those might have been – feminism, politics, religion, your writing, your career, your art. It may be that you have refused to allow your illness to change the course of your life, even if it has altered your priorities. Most important of all, how has the fact of cancer changed your perception of yourself?

As I have already indicated, I do not think that we need to interpret the genre 'essay' as directly autobiographical if we do not wish to do so. Nor are we bound to formal prose discourse. It would be perfectly possible to put the meaning of your own narrative into another shape: fiction, poetry, medical treatise, philosophical dialogue, drama, or as Catherine Arthur has done, into visual art.

This book is a reflection on the meanings of cancer, or on the meanings we can construct for ourselves when we have, or have had, cancer. The women who have written and made this book have all exploited their confrontation with the disease to make their own meanings, or to test the received meanings we find placed upon us as 'cancer victims'. There are no victims here.

This book is unlike other cancer books in that it is, as I had originally desired, 'a thinking about cancer'. The women writing here have chosen very different ways of approaching the illness in its different forms and making sense of their situations. The book is both intensely personal and theoretical. The writers of this book face death with more openness, courage and grim humour than in any other book I have ever read. This is the book I wanted to read when I had cancer. I read feminist texts that suggested I could become a greater, more powerful woman as a result of my experience – all I had to do was turn it to my own advantage and be relentlessly positive – or books that suggested all I needed was God, forgiveness and a good husband. I could not find a book that told me how terrifying it is to die, but that there were still many things I could do, I could say, I could write, that had force and clarity – and that were worth while. This is the book I was looking for, a women's book that was tough-minded, but full of hope.

Patricia Duncker
France, 1996

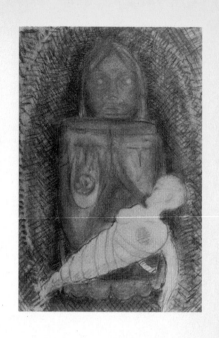

Mother

Introduction
Cathy Read

Cancer is a fact of life for millions of women. It is estimated that one woman in three living in a developed country like the UK will have cancer at some time in her life. Despite improvements in medical technology, there is good evidence that cancer will be with us for some time; there has been little improvement in death rates from most major cancers over the last 30 years.

Although 'cancer' is an umbrella term for some hundred different diseases, the word evokes a common dread. In the *Oxford Encyclopaedic English Dictionary* it is defined both as a 'malignant growth' and 'an evil influence or corruption spreading uncontrollably'. In practice, the evolution of cancer is a complex process which is only partly understood. Put simply, cancer results from damage to genes which control cell growth. For most human cancers, several genetic 'insults' – episodes of damage to the genes which control cell growth – probably have to occur before the normal control mechanisms are overwhelmed and cancer ensues. The genetic insults which contribute to a cancer may be inherited, as for example in hereditary breast cancer, or acquired through exposure to carcinogens in the environment such as radiation, chemical pollution or infectious organisms. Although small amounts of damage occur repeatedly within our genes, particularly when cells are dividing, these are usually rapidly repaired. A fault in the body's gene repair mechanisms, perhaps exacerbated by a deficiency in diet, may also contribute to cancer.

Breast cancer is the most common cancer among women in the world; it killed 560,000 women in 1980 and is predicted to claim the lives of one million women annually by the year 2000. After breast cancer, lung and bowel cancer are the most frequent causes of death from cancer among women in most developed countries. In 1992, 78,900 women died from cancer in the UK; of these 15,220 were due to breast cancer, 12,800 due to lung cancer and 9,780 due to cancers of the colon and rectum (bowel). Cancer of the cervix is the most common form of cancer in women in most developing countries.

There are few signs that the worldwide cancer epidemic is abating. For certain cancers the reverse seems to be true. The incidences of lung cancer and malignant melanoma (skin cancer) among men and women, breast cancer among women and cancer of the prostate and testes among men have increased in many countries over recent decades. These increases appear 'real' and remain even when the ageing population, among whom cancer is more common, has been taken into account. Former US President Nixon launched a 'war against cancer', enshrined in the US National Cancer Act of 1971. The war continues; despite billions of dollars and much hype from cancer charities and the media, death rates from all the major cancers except stomach cancer have shown little improvement in three decades.

This book is a notable addition to a handful of forthright books from the people who really know about cancer. As Felly Nkweto Simmonds tells us with humour and fear, it is all too easy to cross an unseen boundary and suddenly find oneself a 'statistic' in a 'pink plush' waiting room or on a cancer ward. The women who have contributed to this book tell us what numbers on a piece of paper cannot. No woman who has had cancer continues her life unchanged. *Cancer: through the eyes of ten women* shows us in words and images how cancer affects relationships, work, family, sexuality and the meaning women give to their own bodies.

The editors of this volume deliberately sought out an alternative to 'the cancer narrative' where the cancer victim battles it out, love conquers everything and, whether death intervenes or not, there is finally a Great Triumph of the Human Spirit. This collection does not invalidate the experiences of those who genuinely experience cancer in this way. But it looks behind the 'curtain of normality' which is rapidly drawn around many people who are diagnosed with cancer.

Through the eyes of the contributors to this book we are helped to understand the fear, the loss of control, the sense of bereavement at the loss of a breast or other body part, the physical pain and the emotional pain when relationships are thrown into turmoil. Marilyn Hacker says her 'self-betraying body needs to grieve at how hatreds metastasize'. Although many women who have been treated for cancer will share this sentiment, they cannot read it in a medical textbook or a patient information leaflet.

It is important to listen to these voices, and their experience tells us that cancer *is* a feminist issue. Men as well as women get cancer. But a constellation of reasons enable us to approach women's cancer from a feminist perspective. Feminists have a history of empowering themselves in health issues – over the last few decades women around the globe have campaigned hard to assert their right to ownership and control of their own bodies. Women in many countries have achieved control over their fertility, changed antiquated social values and reformed laws on rape, abuse and sexual harrassment, and have begun to demedicalise normal childbirth. Women have worked hard to assert their rights as consumers within male-dominated health services. They have achieved major advances in the amount and quality of information which all patients can expect from healthcare providers, and have established higher standards for 'informed consent' to operations and other medical treatment. The women's cancer movement is a logical continuation of these reforms.

The experience of certain types of cancer is unique to women, particularly cancer of the breast, cervix and ovary. These cancers carry a significance for women because the cancer, and often the treatment, assaults parts of the body which define women as female. When surgery is required, breast cancer involves the most visible assault. The deep sense of loss experienced by some women who undergo mastectomy is related partly to the sexual objectification of breasts in our society, which may leave one-breasted women feeling undesirable, and partly to the way women themselves see their breasts as intimately connected with their fertility and ability to nurture.

Cancer also has a particular relevance for women which reflects their role in society. After a diagnosis of cancer, life takes on an immediacy that demands a change in priorities for many women. Women's relationships often undergo major changes and the experience of cancer may have a profound effect on the way women see themselves. As carers in society, women spend most of their lives nurturing others. Now women who have spent a lifetime giving love to other people have to learn to love themselves.

Survival from cancer varies widely depending on the type and the stage at which it is discovered and treated. For this reason a great deal of effort has been invested in screening programmes to detect pre-cancer or established cancer at an early stage. But while mammography to detect early breast cancer by X-ray diagnosis has been shown to reduce deaths from breast cancer among women aged 50–65 who attend for regular screening, it is now recognised that even if existing screening programmes ran optimally they could only bring about a small reduction in overall deaths from breast cancer.

Screening for cervical cancer has been shown to be effective in the Nordic countries. However, screening in the UK has been troubled with problems of organisation and accountability, and there has been no reduction in the overall number of new cases of invasive cancer of the cervix and only a small reduction in the number of women who die from the disease.

There have also been problems in the UK with access to state-of-the-art cancer services. Cancer treatment in Britain has been described as a 'lottery' where people lucky enough to live near major cancer centres stand a better chance of survival than those treated at some non-specialist centres. The Government has now intervened and cancer services are currently being overhauled and concentrated in designated centres with special expertise. This book illustrates the uneven experiences of women at the hands of the health services of three countries: the UK, France and the US.

Advances in technology are promising us a 'golden age' for cancer treatment in the future. We can expect screening and therefore earlier detection for many more cancers, including cancers of the ovary and bowel. More sophisticated drugs and methods of delivering drugs and radiotherapy to cancer sites will enable cancer to be treated more effectively without involving side-effects throughout the body. Novel treatments including gene therapy will be used to prevent and treat many common cancers. Women who have become politicised about cancer are asking whether the best cure for cancer is to wait for the 'golden age' to arrive.

Most cancers could be prevented or detected earlier with knowledge that is already available. It is estimated that some 80–90 per cent of cancers in northern industrialised countries are caused by environmental or 'lifestyle' factors. Some of these factors, particularly dietary factors, smoking and physical inactivity, also contribute to other chronic diseases including osteoporosis, coronary heart disease and some types of diabetes. Smoking is still a major, avoidable cause of many cancers, including 80–90 per cent of lung cancers and a proportion of deaths from many other types of cancer including cancer of the cervix. In Scotland and some parts of Northern England, death from lung cancer has overtaken death from breast cancer as the commonest cause of cancer death among women.

There is evidence that the 'fast food' diets increasingly consumed throughout Western countries may be related to over 15 different cancers including those of the bowel, lung, mouth, oesophagus and breast. The typical Western diet is characterized by a high fat and calorie content and a lack of fresh fruits, vegetables, fibre and whole grains. Over the last few decades levels of physical activity have declined steeply due to the increased use of labour-saving devices at home and work, increased use of cars and the increased popularity of less active leisure pursuits such as watching television and using home computers. The World Health Organisation has pointed out that physical inactivity may contribute to cancers of the colon, lung, breast and prostate.

Environmental pollution also contributes to the current burden of cancer. Although chemical pollutants and radiation have been underestimated as causes of cancer in the past, they are now coming under greater scrutiny. Chemicals in the environment which mimic oestrogen may be contributing to several 'hormonal' cancers including breast cancer in women and testicular cancer in men. Many of the chemicals under investigation are contained in everyday household items such as plastics, food wrappings and detergents, so they are almost impossible to avoid. Electromagnetic radiation from power lines has been linked with leukaemia and is being investigated for links with other cancers including brain cancer.

Governments recognise the role of environmental factors including diet and have drawn up policy objectives to reduce ill health and deaths from cancer. These objectives are set out by the UK Government in 'The Health of the Nation', and the Committee of European Cancer Experts has drawn up a European code against cancer which advises on preventive measures people can take to avoid it. But as long as we live in societies which foster a cancer culture – where people are repeatedly exposed to factors which may initiate or promote cancer in the course of everyday life – advice on cancer prevention aimed at individuals is likely to have limited impact. By implication, it says that by being 'good' people can largely avoid cancer, while in reality many of the factors which influence cancer are beyond most people's immediate control. There is, for example, a connection between poverty and cancer. In the UK, women in the lowest economic bracket are three times more likely to die of cancer of the cervix than those in the highest group. And while deaths from lung cancer have fallen among women from the wealthiest classes, they have risen among the poorest women.

Government objectives to reduce cancer need to be backed by political action. For example, the UK Government hopes to cut the number of people who smoke (and thereby reduce deaths from lung cancer) by a third by the year 2000. However, it has failed to ban tobacco advertising or reduce consumption by steep price increases. Surveys show that children smoke the brands that are most heavily advertised, and it is estimated that the government receives some £70 million a year in tax on cigarettes sold illegally to children under the age of 16.

Against this background, the women's cancer movement pioneered in the northeastern United States is an important focus for change. The testimonies of women with cancer have already begun to change the agenda for breast cancer. Vigorous campaigning by the women-led National Breast Cancer Coalition in the US increased government spending from $90 million to $500 million on breast cancer services and research in just five years. The US experience is being repeated elsewhere. In 1995 a National Breast Cancer Coalition was launched in the UK, with the three major aims of improving access to state-of-the-art treatment for all women, increasing Government spending on research (including causes, prevention and quality of life issues), and involving women in decisions about breast cancer issues.

These women-led reforms represent genuine progress. There is a growing recognition that science and medicine cannot solve society's problems so long as they work in isolation. Scientific problems such as cancer have a social dimension, and the experiences and opinions of people who have cancer are as valid as those of scientists and doctors. *Cancer: through the eyes of ten women* gives all of us a different view of cancer.

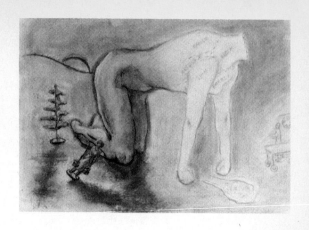

Mrs Beeton's Cow

Conquering Heroes:
The Politics of Cancer Narratives
Jackie Stacey
For Sahra

I

Accounts of cancer always tell stories. Those who write them offer recognizable narratives of diagnosis, of treatment and of prognosis. Those who read them often do so in search of the comforting hope of survival. Faced with a sudden change in the story of their lives following a cancer diagnosis, many rehearse the possible trajectories which now present themselves through the stories of those who have been there before them.

There are books written by doctors about 'the facts' you need to know: these tell of the different types of cancer, the typical prognoses and the likely treatments and their side-effects.[1] There are books written by alternative practitioners encouraging a holistic approach to the disease, advising on diet, therapy and a change of lifestyle.[2] There are books written by spiritual 'evangelists' who write of cancer as an opportunity for salvation.[3]

There are also, of course, books written by patients, or their friends and relatives, which offer personal accounts of the experience of living

I

with (and sometimes dying of) cancer. If the person with cancer has lived to tell the tale, the story is often of a heroic struggle against adversity. Pitting life against death and drawing on all possible resources, the patient moves from victim to survivor and 'triumphs over the tragedy' which has unexpectedly threated his or her life. These are often stories of transformation in which the negative physical affliction becomes a positive source of self-knowledge. The person who has faced death and has recognized the limits of human mortality, and yet lives on, now benefits from a new-found wisdom. Accepting the fragility of life itself, the cancer survivor sees things others are not brave enough to face, or appreciates things others are too busy to notice (or so the story goes). Cancer offers the chance to reassess. It allows the person to pause and to re-evaluate life: having cancer teaches us that life may be shorter than we think and that it may be time to decide to live it differently.[4] These are the kinds of wisdoms which we read and reread in popular accounts of surviving cancer.

If, on the other hand, the person with cancer dies, the story told is one of loss and of pain, but also a celebration of courage and dignity. It may be written by friends, lovers or relatives. Stories of pointlessly shortened lives, lost opportunities, or of medical or industrial malpractice or ineptitude warn others to avoid a similar fate; the late diagnosis, the misread X-ray or the high levels of radiation near nuclear power stations are among the motivations for authors to tell these types of stories.[5] Few write (or publish) accounts which tell only of disaster and depression, suffering and unbearable loss. There is always room for heroism in tragedy, and many stories offer accounts of stoicism and of a fighting spirit, documenting the triumphs along the way, even in the event of death.[6]

The market for books about cancer is enormous. Books about cancer are not hard to find; in fact, they are hard to avoid. Once the news has been broken, books about cancer surface from all directions: they are on every friend's bookshelf, in every shop window. A veritable *cancer subculture* proves to have been thriving, but, like so many others, it remains invisible until it becomes relevant and then, as if by magic, it seems suddenly all-pervasive. For many people with cancer these books are the starting point of coming to terms with their diagnosis. They are read in the hope of finding a story that fits, of finding a story that offers hope, of even finding a story that ends happily. They are also read for information about the disease or about the treatment: some offer the chance to learn the language of oncology, to understand the principles of chemotherapy or radiotherapy; others educate their readers on the workings of the immune system, the anti-cancer diet or the negative effects of stress on the body. Read all of them and you can become an expert in your field, an expert on your particular disease, *an expert on yourself*.

The most rapidly expanding strand of the market currently is what I call *self-health* cancer books. These books combine aspects of alternative medicine with ideas from the therapeutic cultures of self-help. Typically they invite readers to consider certain changes in their physical and emotional lifestyle in order to realise why they got ill and to begin their recovery. The solution lies within individuals and their determination to conquer the parts of themselves that might have caused their cancer. Invariably those with cancer are called upon to exercise mind over matter, to take charge of their body through diet, meditation, therapy and self-acceptance, to become heroes of their own personal narratives and the authors of their new life scripts. These books can be found in their dozens among the growing number of health and fitness/self-development/New Age and spirituality sections of highstreet bookstores and the publications for sale in health food shops.

Given the changes in health cultures in 1990s Britain, the proliferation of a market of self-health cancer books is hardly surprising. The growth in self-health cultures clearly marks out a sense of dissatisfaction with conventional biomedicine. Specific complaints about its patronizing and alienating practices towards patients and discrimination on the basis of gender, class, ethnicity and sexuality combine with a more general disillusionment with scientific and medical expertise. Increasingly the cynicism about Western science as the great liberator and leading force in 'developing' the rest of the world has permeated our popular imagination. While we continue to use biomedicine, we also worry about the certainties its experts promise us, and we are more and more aware of its iatrogenic (disease-producing) effects.

But the growing criticism of conventional medicine is not the only significant factor in the rise in popularity of self-health. As the British Government's cuts in public health provision become the source of endless stories in everyday life (patients returned home prematurely after surgery, beds not available for emergencies, nurses' threats of unprecedented industrial action signalling intense desperation and frustration), people are increasingly encouraged to look elsewhere for reassurances. The introduction of internal markets into the National Health Service in Britain through the National Health Service and Community Care Act (implemented on 1 April 1991) fundamentally changed the system's principles of organization and management, placing health firmly within a world of competition and consumerism.[7] In these emergent health cultures, where the language of the market has come to dominate ideas about health provision, the scope for appealing to individuals to take charge of their health is ever-widening. As the National Health Service no longer guarantees to provide the patient care necessary, the responsibility increasingly shifts elsewhere. As well as expecting 'families' (read women) to do more unpaid caring,[8] there is also a growing imperative for the 'individual' to take responsibility for his or her own health. This is perhaps the most glaring overlap between some of the cultures of self-health and the Thatcherite legacy of the cult of the individual. In the marketization of public sector areas such as health, there has been a shift in responsibility (and thus funding) that encourages us to 'heal ourselves'. The market for cancer books expands as beliefs about self-health capture our imaginations.

II

My own response to being diagnosed with cancer was to read as much as I could about the subject. I borrowed and bought as many books as possible – biomedical, self-health, personal narratives. I sent off to cancer charities for leaflets and phoned helplines for advice. I spent days and weeks, and eventually months, reading about cancer and how to get rid of it. Following the typical pattern of an academic reaction to a problem, my illness quickly became a research project. While I was still in hospital, friends researched the details of the rare kind of cancer I had, since it did not appear in many of the standard accounts. What characterized the cancer I had, and how did it spread? What were my chances and what treatments should I expect? Medical libraries were consulted and bookshops were searched to find the maximum amount of information for my purpose.

This desire for knowledge was clearly a bid for control at the very moment it had been taken away from me. It was also an instrumental use of the academic skills of my world and a way of making the alienating medical world, in which I had suddenly found myself, more familiar and more manageable. Unlike many other people with cancer who do not have my educational advantages, I did have a powerful set of resources to draw upon. Turning the disease into a research project channelled my otherwise overwhelming fear and panic. The desire for information, and the confidence to access it, are often both the privilege of those with certain educational histories, race and class backgrounds and belong to a new generation of what I call *participatory patients*. On the whole, people of my parents' generation, for example, are far less inclined to be put in the picture. They are often happier to leave it to the medical experts and to avoid the burdens and responsibilities such knowledge might demand. But those of us who have been influenced by the information cultures of the last 20 years are more susceptible to the desire to know and to the fantasy that knowledge is power. We are encouraged to seek out information about ourselves with an obsessive curiosity. In my own case, in the context of complete ignorance about my illness I welcomed any new details about my condition.

But the information proved inseparable from the stories: other people's stories, and then very quickly, my own. As the pieces fitted together, a story began to take shape. First the cancer was named. I had

had (and at that time, possibly still had) a teratoma: more specifically, an endodermal sinus tumour, a malignant growth originating in an egg cell in my ovary (it still seems unlikely). Then the tumour type was described: large (the size of a melon), fast-growing, mono-lateral (one-sided). With this information, memory traces were rearranged to produce a retrospective account of the illness: Passing sensations that I had barely registered at the time now took on enormous significance as signs of a life-threatening disease which had been quietly present in my body. The narrative that emerged gradually organized physical sensations into a temporal sequence with a causative effect. Looking back, the abdominal bloating seemed obvious, the pressure on the bladder at night an unquestionable symptom. These almost negligible manifestations were rewritten as the crucial early signs of the disease.

The more recent and much more dramatic physical symptoms are then also rationalized within this pathological trajectory: I am told that the abdominal pain was caused by the tumour rupturing and bleeding into the abdominal cavity, causing the effects of peritonitis. The puzzling events of the first few days of illness are given narrative coherence, and recent conversations and advice take on new meaning in the light of the seriousness of the diagnosis. The doctor who did not insist on immediate surgery now looks to have been somewhat negligent: his permission to wait six weeks for surgery, which seemed a god-send at the time, is condemned as incompetent. His female superior, who finally made a correct diagnosis and insisted on emergency surgery on a Sunday, becomes an angel rescuing me from imminent danger.

The narrative of my body continued to be rewritten in this way with each new stage. As I lay recovering from surgery, I tried to find out what had been removed apart from the tumour. They had taken out the tumour and also the fallopian tube and the ovary on the right side. Overnight my identity was reinvented: I was now a cancer patient; or was I? I was told the disease might or might not still be present in my body. It might or might not return. Since the tumour had ruptured, some malignant cells might have been left behind and therefore chemotherapy might be necessary. Weekly tests would tell.

It soon became the story of uncertainty. Impossible to predict the future, because the present situation might change at any moment. Next year might be beyond reach. Next month I might be back at work or in hospital having chemotherapy. According to the statistics, I reminded myself, I had an 80-90 per cent chance of recovery. A hopeful prognosis by all accounts.

Illness thus becomes a narrative very rapidly. Some sense is sought of time and sequence, sense for others and for oneself. The past confusion is explained; the present situation requires a story (I struggle to offer a coherent answer to the question 'what has happened?'); the future presents the possibility of terrifying resolutions (what are my chances of survival?) Only a little information is necessary and the narrative structuring begins: linearity, cause and effect and possible closures present themselves almost automatically. Decide on the name of the disease, explain a few symptoms, predict the outcome and the story is practically written. Indeed, the genres of medical knowledge are organized around just such temporal trajectories: diagnosis, treatment and prognosis are in some ways just other names for the different stages of the story.

The usual temporal sequencing is both disrupted and reimposed in the search for order, reason and predictability. The past must now be re-imagined and re-scripted. Life, it has turned out, was not what it appeared to be. The present is not the imagined future it once was. And as for the future, it is suddenly compressed into the most frightening of time scales, previously unimaginable. In the light of the cancer diagnosis, the recent past must be re-examined for clues to this newly-revealed deception. The body thus becomes the site of a narrative teleology that demands a re-telling.

Given the demands of this new bodily evidence, I found myself inventing new stories about myself. If such an illness had been present the whole summer (perhaps longer?), what sense could be made of the memories of those idyllic months? 'But you looked so well' became the incredulous refrain of friends and family. Perhaps these memories themselves were simply the nostalgic product of the loss (of good health). Were those remembered weeks in which I had felt 'better than I had for years' simply a retrospective reinvention at a time of danger and threat, feelings of a golden age that emerge in the face of mortality? The old narratives struggle against the pressures of the new, which have the advantage of immediacy, physical presence and, indeed, medical emergency. The body tells a new story and so demands a reinterpretation of recent life history. Is the body no longer to be trusted? Should it ever have been? Why has it withheld such crucial evidence? Whose side is it on, anyway?

In the light of the cancer diagnosis, these new narratives of the body re-script the story of my life with ruthless editorial authority. While the mind had been full of stories of life, the body had been planning another story: the threat of death. How should my life be imagined in such an unexpected context? Can the self be reinvented to cope with the shock? What kind of person does not know they have cancer? What kind of body hides the evidence so effectively? And what kind of disease could disguise itself so skilfully? I had thought I was aware of my body and its complaints. I had assumed that I could read the corporeal codes. I was body literate. I could see the signs. I knew if protest was taking place. I had learned to 'listen to my body' over the years. But the shock of this diagnosis suggested that all was not what it seemed: the healthy body hosted deadly disease; the smooth surface concealed a large malignant tumour. My energy for life that summer had been matched by another: the prolific growth of a malignant disease. How could they have pulled in such opposite directions with the same enthusiasm? Competing agendas and conflicting trajectories: whose authority would win out?

Given these sudden changes, I had to find new ways of writing the story of my life. I had to consider the story of my death with an unprecedented urgency. Before my diagnosis I had harboured a clichéd (and yet barely articulated) fantasy that I would live until my early eighties and would die suddenly, but peacefully, in my armchair. Not that I spent much time planning that far ahead, but following such a diagnosis many semi-conscious projections that inform our sense of ourselves surface and take on a more definite shape. Moreover, the shock of the diagnosis not only produces a rapid series of re-narra-tivizations, but also illuminates the extent to which all kinds of narra-tives have quietly and unconsciously structured our imagination up until the present time.

When I was first diagnosed with cancer my initial shock placed me outside the narrative of my own life, watching it as if it were on film (a predictable visual manifestation of the cliché 'and her life appeared before her' for someone who teaches film and media studies). I felt certain someone had got the story wrong; this was not how it was supposed to go. The first reel of the film had finished and the rest of my life, already recorded on the second reel which lay next to the projector, ready and waiting to be screened, had been forgotten. There was at least another half to go. The whole episode felt as if it were someone else's script, not mine. The denial of the powerlessness produced a cinematic trope which seemed to offer a guarantee of narrative certainty and predictability: there should be a whole second half still to show.

At the next stage, chemotherapy did in fact prove necessary: four doses of it over the course of three months. It seemed to work. It was followed by weekly, then monthly, then quarterly and now six-monthly tests. But there are few real certainties with cancer narratives and so many possible complications that it is hard to know when to breathe that sigh of relief that puts the illness in the past. Some three years on, I finally became confident enough to speak about it in the past tense. For many months I had used the present perfect tense to describe my situation, 'I have had cancer' – it started in the past and may be continuing in the present (as the grammar books put it). To have used the present tense, 'I have cancer,' seemed too pessimistic, since I hoped I did not any more. But while writing this piece I had a letter following my annual scan telling me that a report had been sent to my consultant warning that 'the uterus looks bulky and there's a suggestion of a cyst on the other ovary.' With further investigation this proved to be a false alarm and I was 'reassured' that the radiologist had 'overread the image'. There was nothing to worry about. Thus, although when I first drafted this I felt as if my particular cancer story was almost over, this recent episode only serves to underline the ways in which cancer narratives refuse to offer the reassurances of complete resolution. I have rewritten this piece in at least two or three different tenses. Its final version remains (appropriately perhaps) a mixture.

Few cancers are considered completely curable, and consultants hedge around such absolutes in their conversations with patients. I am much more fortunate than many insofar as there is a five-year threshold for teratoma patients, the crossing of which promises the all-clear. There is still another year or so of tests, although I am told that I am on much safer ground these days. But there are so many variables with cancer and its treatments. Some chemotherapy can cause long-term side-effects. In my case, while the teratoma may remain banished, I have been told that the chemotherapy may cause leukaemia in 15 to 20 years' time – though it may not, of course. Added to such prospects is the litany of so-called 'side-effects' of chemotherapy. These continue to change my self-image, aspirations and the stories I tell myself and others about my life and the kind of person I am in the world.

As the distance between the initial diagnosis and my present state of relatively 'good health' grows, my memories of the experience become more muddled, but the narrativization of certain events increasingly solidifies. As the stories have taken shape a new teleology has been produced. Present self has begun to connect to past and future selves through narrative structures that have placed a meaning where there had been only confusion. I now have my own stories of diagnosis, of treatments, of prognosis and, indeed (hopefully), of survival. The narrative follows one of the typical trajectories: crisis, rescue and recovery. Despite resistance to the absolutes of closure, I still push my own particular story in that desirable direction. Although it is not over yet, the whole episode can now be represented in a series of narratives: when people ask about the experience, I have plenty of stories to tell.

III

Cultural narratives in general offer reassuring accounts of problems which have resolutions. Be it in self-health cancer books, Hollywood cinema, or Shakespeare's plays, narratives move from problem to resolution with some sense of predictability and comforting repetition. There may be hold-ups, detours or unexpected twists along the way (indeed, this is par for the course), but on the whole the stories that surround us are those whose riddles are solved, whose enigmas are understood, whose villains are destroyed and whose lost order is restored. Narrative offers a way of ordering events and assigning roles; it gives temporal continuity and spatial coherence. The term 'narrative' draws attention to the story as convention and highlights the cultural forms of its typical patterns.[9] The repeated use of particular structures across a range of genres suggests that narratives offer fantasies of the triumph of good over evil and of order over confusion. Thus a common formula in popular culture is as follows: the stasis of a character, a community or a nation is threatened by corruption or invasion from outside (or from an enemy within); this produces chaos and yet offers the chance to explore the threat to its limits before it is eradicated; the reassuring narrative closure re-establishes order; this is often a new and better order than that disrupted in the first place.[10]

In popular cultural narratives it is usually the *male* protagonist who takes a number of risks in the name of truth, justice, morality or love, and in overcoming the negative forces in favour of these principles he (or sometimes she) achieves a heroic stature which we might all admire or even aspire to. These masculine heroes offer fantasies of invincibility. They are the larger-than-life ego ideals who shape our hopes. Their bodies are impenetrable and their boundaries are immutable. Their force is indestructible and their certainty undiminishable. Being on their side, we might imagine ourselves to be the agents of history; identifying with their power, we believe ourselves to control our destinies. These are the heroes who enable us to trust ourselves, to trust our judgment, to know we are right. We too can be omnipotent; we can take charge. These have been the (enviable?) forms of masculine heroism that have been challenged by recent feminist cultural criticism. Those of us engaged in such debates may become aware of the power of such fantasies of transcendence at precisely the moments in our lives when we are forced to reshape our self-narrativization.

Stories about illness are an intensification of the way in which we generally understand our lives through narrative. The experience of cancer may bring these narrative processes into particularly sharp focus, but in many ways it only makes explicit the importance of narratives in the construction of the self in contemporary culture.[11] We have stories about our childhood, a mixture of our memories and the family favourites we have heard repeatedly. We tell stories about our relationships, both successful and otherwise. We relate our (public and private) stories about who we are and what makes us special or different from the next person.[12] We have projected stories about whom we might become in the future through relationships, paid work, parenthood, sport and leisure activities and so on. When something unexpected occurs, such as illness, the scripts need rewriting, but normally the shock of the experience can be partly absorbed by the telling of a new story. The clash with the previous stories gradually loses its impact as the experience is integrated as a narrative feature in its own right. Life before and after illness; life before and after a baby; life before and after a partner; life before and after (a) death.

In contemporary Western culture we are encouraged to think of our lives as coherent stories of success, progress and movement forward. Loss and failure have their place, but only as part of a broader picture of ascendence. The steady upward curve is the favoured contour. Different relationships to material and psychic privileges offer inequitable resources for the fulfilment of plans and ambitions, and dreams may seem more realizable for some than for others. In a society so obsessed with its own progress and improvement, it is almost impossible for us to avoid the pull of such narratives. In the face of crisis, another story begins and with the power of retrospection the past is rewritten for the needs of the present and hopes for the future.

But the power of narrative is not always enough to pull us through. With its demand for spatial and temporal coherence, for linear sequence and for closure and resolution, conventional narrative structure cannot necessarily contain the demands of a changing world. Autobiographical accounts of people with HIV and AIDS, for example, have begun to reshape the contours of narrative.[13] What sense can be made of the temporal continuity that characterizes the autobiographical form for the writer with AIDS, whose only imaginable future promises bodily decline? And what kind of new spatial dimensions need to be invented to accommodate the imagined identities of those living with the insecurities of borrowed time? AIDS narratives might thus be said to have put pressure on the structures of conventional genres of story-telling. For some, it is argued, there is now a general anxiety about the narrative meaning of time in a culture where knowledge about AIDS has thrown into question conventional temporal securities and predictable trajectories of self-development.[14]

Cancer, too, threatens to rob us of our dreams of the future. But the uncertainties it generates are typically transformed into the hope of a return to familiar narrative structures. For some, the diagnosis of cancer may be as final as the diagnosis of being HIV positive (though the possibility of a cure for both may nevertheless perform a hope function). But for others the triumph-over-tragedy story offers a structure for an imagined future. Cancer and AIDS both have highly unpredictable prognostic patterns, but at the moment, at least, some forms of cancer are considered curable if caught at an early enough stage. The temporal expectations of the subject of cancer are thus thrown into question, but not necessarily radically fractured as they are said to be for those writing about their experiences of HIV and AIDS.

Cancer does not really invade the body as such, but rather reproduces itself from the inside. Malignant growths secretly proliferate. Like the monster of screen horror, cancer threatens bodily order and takes over the body's regulating systems. Horror films often tell tales of the conquering of monsters. Invaders from outside (and increasingly from inside) threaten the order of human society and must be exterminated in the name of civilization as we know it.[15] More often than not the monstrous threat invades the body. Occupied by an alien force or physical presence, the innocent human victims lose control of the body and its functions.[16] Be its protagonists vampires, ghouls, or monsters from outer space, the horror narrative explores the boundaries between human and non-human, between life and death and between self and other. Its resolution requires the expulsion of the alien from the physical and social body it threatens and the re-establishment of human order and stability. The heroes (the good scientists, the decent citizens, the protective fathers and husbands – and very occasionally the Sigourney Weavers) fight the monster to its death and return the rule of law to its rightful supremacy.[17]

Stories of surviving cancer fit easily into these patterns of a journey from chaos to control.[18] They combine the masculine heroics of such narratives with the feminine suffering and sacrifice of melodramas. The narrative structure lends itself well to such masculine heroic epics combined with the emotional intensity of the more feminine 'triumph over tragedy' genre. There is the meta-narrative of the fight against cancer in general, accompanied by the micro-narratives of the emotional episodes along the way. While the books I read varied a great deal, stories of heroes, victims and villains were never far away. The crisis-rescue-recovery formulation positions the hero against the disease in a life-and-death battle. The hero usually has truth, goodness and the pursuit of knowledge on his/her side. People who survive cancer are transformed from feminized victim to masculinized hero in the narrative re-telling of individual triumph.

The narrativization of the struggle against cancer pervades all representations of the disease. In biomedical accounts it is scientific progress that is heroised: science will produce the cure for cancer (eventually). So often it is the heroic men of medicine who are represented as victors; so often they save women from the horrors of their bodies. Cancer is commonly seen as the cells in chaos, the body out of control, governed only by the rules of outlaws. Medical science, personified in the figure of the doctor, brings the chance of rationalization, the promise of order.

Cancer is a disease against which Western science has long waged battle. We are told that science is winning.[19] Through the progress of scientific discovery and the pursuit of more and more knowledge, the fantasy of ultimate control is offered: with enough time and money, cures will be found. Each new discovery offers the chance of cracking the code, of solving the cancerous riddle which has brought death to so many. Genetics, the information science, is the latest in a long line of disciplinary developments which promise to stretch the limits of knowledge and give us the power to defy the disease. We now read of the 'oncogene': the final frontier? If the gene can be isolated, surely a cure is in sight?[20]

In my own research on the teratoma, I read about how it used to be one of the most fatal cancers, killing its victims within 18 months, its unusually fast-growing cells spreading through the body like wild fire. In the 1990s, however, it is one of the most treatable cancers; the discovery of a particular chemotherapy cocktail, which acts effectively on such rapidly-dividing cells, has brought an *almost* guaranteed promise of a cure. Bleomycin, Etopicide and Cisplatinum provide the magic formula in most cases. From the 'worst' to the 'best' kind of cancer in 15 years. Thank God for scientific discovery; I could feel myself inclining towards hero worship. Faced with a teratoma which might devour my body within the next year, medical science became the welcome rescuer. The medical accounts of the teratoma exemplified the success of the scientific project, of the steady upward curve, the ever-expanding boundaries of scientific knowledge. Medical science had discovered a cure and I would be saved.

The appeal of the masculine hero narratives of science cannot be overestimated. Trust the doctors, they know best. Your body becomes the battleground between good science and bad disease. If you give yourself up to the medical establishment's wisdom and follow their instructions you stand the best chance. Many (though by no means all) medical staff show little tolerance for patients who do otherwise. Indeed, some warn that you ignore their instructions at your peril. One woman in her first-person account of breast cancer treatment claims that she was labelled a 'non-cooperator' and a 'militant' by hospital staff, and was warned of the consequences.[21] Medical experts are there to make the decisions for you (or so we might suppose) and we can hope they will shoulder the responsibility for the narrative outcome, for it is *their* job to do so. Of course, even the most conventional of biomedics would agree that a positive patient is preferable, but beyond this the patient has little determining effect on the direction of the story. The biomedics alone are the narrators, perhaps even the authors.

In the alternative medical and self-health accounts, by contrast, it is the patient (probably with the help of the practitioner or therapist) who becomes the hero. With the correct guidance, the cancer patient can discover a new self, a true self, an Ur-self (or original self); you are invited to 'become who you are', or rather, to become 'who you should have been'. With suitable monitoring, this new self can be maintained as a *defended self*: the fantasy of masculine invincibility surfaces again.[22] Although the patient is positioned differently in these accounts, the structure of the narrative is very similar to those within biomedicine. The typical story is of the patient who is unexpectedly diagnosed as having cancer, who plummets to the depths of despair, who reassesses his or her values and the meaning of life and who rises phoenix-like from the experience a new and better person. Having given the patient the chance of a new start in life, cancer in retrospect feels like a blessing in disguise, we are told. Indeed, with the wisdom of hindsight, the person who has now overcome the threat of cancer is able to see how the cancer was an integral part of his or her previous follies, now abandoned. Cancer is interpreted as a metaphor for the self-destructive lifestyle that has since been rejected. The tumour eating away at the body is seen as a sign of unhappiness, distress or indeed, dis-ease. Through diet, relaxation, emotional expression and various kinds of alternative medicine and self-help, patients cure themselves of cancer and go on to lead happier lives than before. And, moreover, they live to tell the tale.

Cancer is thus constructed as a monstrous physical manifestation of other problems: these may be the problems of modernity (pollution, workaholism, chemicals and so on); or of a repressive and repressed culture which cannot deal with emotional life and prefers instead to be governed by rationality and the intellect. In both respects, masculine values *seem* to be under attack. However, the extent to which the so-called self-help alternatives to conventional, masculinized culture really introduce new ways of conceptualizing the self in the world is debatable. In particular, the forms of individualism produced within these alternative accounts definitely have a gendered appeal in terms of their heroic forms, not to mention their potential complicity with emergent and established forms of enterprise culture.[23] An ambivalence towards certain kinds of self-health approaches to cancer was my own starting point for a detailed analysis of the discourses which form the basis for their 'truth claims'.

The narrative structure of many self-health accounts of cancer follows the traditional pattern of the hero fighting an unexpected or unwelcome enemy. The shock of this disruption, however, is followed by the relief of the successful battle against it and the restoration of order following its exclusion. Conflict between good and evil is thus still at the heart of this kind of cancer narrative. The person with cancer is offered the opportunity to achieve heroism through bravery, fortitude and strength of will. Having faced death and survived, the heroes of those narratives are good and wise and true to themselves. These are stories of individual heroes. Social identities, such as race, class or gender, are barely mentioned and instead the focus is on the extraordinary qualities of the individuals: their exceptionalism. Indeed, it is often precisely individuality that is at stake in the healing process. Through the experience of the disease and the fight against it, these people become heroes by discovering their uniqueness and individuality. This is the true merit of the trauma: the chance to find oneself.

IV

It is impossible to have cancer and not to be seduced by the power of such cultural narratives. Part of the appeal of books about cancer is their promise of a compelling narrative: the key elements are bound to be present – life and death, a conflict, heroism, and the heightened emotional intensity that characterizes the best of all stories.

It is tempting to write such a story here, and it would be easy to do so. I could include all the ingredients of the classic 'triumph over tragedy' genre: starting at the beginning, there was the shock of it all – so young for cancer and so fit (or so we thought); moving through the numerous twists in the middle – the 'misdiagnosis', the suspense of the weekly tests, 12 weeks of improvement followed by a relapse, the horror of the treatment, the relief when it ended; and moving finally towards the available closures – the hair growing back, returning to work, coming to terms with my new physical limits, crossing the two-year threshold, having survived. I could write the story of a hero's successful struggle and you could read about it. It might satisfy my need for recognition, for external validation, or for the experience to become a distant narrative; it might satisfy some readers' curiosity to know about this cancer from a safe distance, to be glad it was not their fate, or, for those who have been there too (or who fear they may be next) it might offer the chance to compare notes or to prepare themselves.

But what is not told through such heroic narratives? What does their linear form exclude? What cannot be restored with closure? Where is the continued chaos and disorder in such accounts? Where is the forgotten pain? Stories of progress and rationality are tempting, but perpetuate the illusion of life as a steady upward learning curve in which all crises have a profound meaning and show that 'God is working His purpose out.' Such mythologies encourage us to believe that suffering makes us wiser, and serve to heroise those who suffer the most. They leave no room for the futility of the pain and the arbitrariness of disease, the unbearable pointlessness of suffering. They cover the absences, the amnesia and the gaps in the story. They iron out the competing accounts, the multiple meanings, the lack of meaning. They offer the promise of delivering the 'truth' about the illness: the essence of self and the essence of the disease brought together in a tightly structured account. They offer fantasies of power and control through the narrative rationalizations of progress and improvement. The universality of human goodness and the transcendence of the suffering cancer patient fit easily into familiar narrative structures of good triumphing over evil.

Heroic cancer narratives also reproduce the conventional privileging of the triumphs of a few at the expense of the majority. The lucky ones (though they are never called that) are celebrated, while the rest suffer defeat. The heroes of cancer are represented as special people, as unique individuals, as better than the rest: Isn't she brave? Isn't he wonderful? They are supposed to have died five years ago but have since climbed every mountain; they did not notice the treatment and kept working while others fell around them; they fought until the end but then died gracefully. And what of the others? What of those who declined rapidly, who cried with fear and terror in the face of death, who continue to be haunted by the threat of the cancer returning or for whom there is no 'hope'? What of those who do not smile bravely? In the success/failure binarisms of hero narratives these people can only be seen as failures. Sadly, they did not rise to heroic status. They may not feel wiser now, but more confused, bitter, cheated. Theirs may not have been the story of discovering the generosity of the human spirit, of the bountiful goodness of friends and family. Perhaps they discovered new depths of loneliness and depression, or felt betrayed and abandoned by those they relied upon. What if everyone around them was not so wonderful?[24] And what if there was no one around, wonderful or not? In the heroic cancer narratives written in so many books, these stories are left untold.

I thus return to the political questions raised by cultural narratives. The dangers of the success story hover above me as I write, and yet narration is impossible to avoid and brings irreplaceable comforts to many. Is narrative possible, then, without these dubious forms of heroism? Might we rescue certain kinds of story-telling from their more conservative tendencies? Or should we even consider the more positive dimensions of heroism itself: cannot it also inspire and lead the way? After all, it offers structure and purpose to a sense of self shattered by fear and panic. If I found comfort in the processes of narration and if this gave my overwhelming fear a direction, why seek to deny others such an opportunity? Is not the process of telling one's story and of being heard significant and restorative in itself?

Cancer (and other) support groups testify to the powers of affirmation and 'witnessing'.[25] The feeling that 'someone has heard my story', and that it is legitimate to want to tell that story, calms the psyche. It can offer the necessary reassurance at a time of crisis or trauma, or the route out of it retrospectively. The feeling of not being alone that is offered by narrative identifications has increasingly become a central component of 'cancer patient culture'. Informal networks of people eager to share their stories and to hear those of others have sprung up all over the country. There are literally hundreds of such groups. While the person with cancer is ill, his or her peers are likely to be at school or at work and life goes on with its routine freneticism. Often there is only one child in a class with leukaemia, only one lecturer with a teratoma (though women in their fifties with breast cancer may find many friends and colleagues in the same boat). Relating one's story may offer support, comfort and reassurance. It may help people to live through the trauma of the illness and the treatment and may help those who are recovering to begin to put the experience into the past tense.

In my own case this sense of isolation seemed especially acute, as the cancer I had was so rare: only one other case in the last five years at the second-largest cancer centre in England where I was being treated. I was constantly told how unusual I was. I was unlikely to meet anyone with the same disease. In addition, my response to the chemotherapy was so acute that I developed endless side-effects which seemed to make me an even rarer case. A teratoma patient had rarely had quite so many side-effects or had these particular side-effects so badly, I was told. For a whole host of reasons, I stood out. Others on my ward were much older than I was. Support groups were typically for an older age group. I was not married with children. I was having a relationship with a woman. I was using a number of alternative treatments against cancer as well as the conventional ones. I did not wear a wig – the only one on the ward without one. So not only did I feel cut off from friends who, for all their generous support, continued in their busy schedules of work and play (as I would have done in their position), but I felt separate from the cancer cultures I found myself unwillingly inhabiting. In this context my story had a certain freakish ring to it: no one else seemed to have been here before.

V

We had chosen the holiday as an end-of-chemotherapy treat. More expensive than we could really afford, but that was part of its appeal. We spent days choosing from hundreds of options: France, Italy, Greece; self-catering, hotel or taverna; the week after the final treatment or later than that? How could you plan a holiday when there were so many variables? The story of the treatment kept changing: five doses, then four; postponed because of side-effects; postponed because of bed shortages. When would I be finished and well enough to travel? No one knew. If the final treatment had not been cancelled, we'd have had to have changed the dates. If I'd readmitted myself when the vomiting wouldn't stop after the fourth treatment, they may have urged me to wait longer. In the midst of this uncertainty, we plumped for a date: we would go on 14 April, for two weeks. Such indulgence. Booked in February as an incentive to get me through it. It helped with visualization: I was on a Greek island in the warmth of the sun, and with the sound of waves to comfort me. I memorized the description of 'Olive Tree Cottages' from the holiday brochure:

> As the road climbs towards the gorge, you can just catch a glimpse of the tiled roofs of the cottage below you, peeping out between green olive trees on the far side of the river bed and framed by the endless blue vistas of the Libyan Sea ... Hidden away round the corner from the main cottage, this

studio ... has french windows from the sleeping area [which] lead out to a cloistered little patio facing west with a shady olive tree to one side. Beyond the patio with its fringe of flowers, shrubs and a gnarled old Carob tree, the land drops away to the dried up river bed, where trees grow in profusion and birds sing joyfully in the sunshine.

This place was chosen because it was away from the main village. If I wanted to, I could hide away from the usual people-watching of holiday chic and enjoy the privacy of seclusion. And of course as I walked down the main street of Paleachora in Crete, people stared. They always stare, but on this holiday they stared a lot. Not surprising, really. I had lost eyebrows, eyelashes and hair, and that does give a person an unusual look. I wore a scarf or a hat in public, but I did look different. Certainly no one else looked like me. That is, until two women walked towards us, one of whom wore a pale blue headscarf wound round in a recognizable turban style. She also had that rather uncannily naked look of someone with no eyebrows or eyelashes. She looked completely familiar and yet totally unfamiliar at the same time. Did I do a double-take, or did I just imagine I did? How obvious was the shock in my expression? In a typically English way we passed each other without acknowledgement. With apparent indifference to each other's recent histories, we walked on politely.

This youngish woman (in her twenties?) who bore a strange resemblance to me had suddenly appeared as my mirror image in a street in a small Greek village. I could not wait to get back to the flat and tell all. I wished I had spoken to her, but what would I have said? 'Excuse me, are you English and have you had chemotherapy? That's strange, so have I.' It seemed absurd, but also foolish not to. We would probably never see each other again. She could have been on a day trip, or might have disappeared into a large hotel far away from where I was staying. Instead of these more likely options, however, I saw the same woman again: this time not in the public thoroughfare of the village but in the relative privacy of the entrance to Olive Tree Cottages. Obviously returning from a mountain hike, she and her companion went in through the front door of the other self-catering studio flat. There were only three apartments in this terrace; between us we occupied two of them. Next-door-but-one: this was too much to bear; I *had* to go and speak to her. My whole body buzzed with the excitement of coincidence.

Keen to reclaim my body again after months of sickness, I was driven by a desire to get fit like never before. Walking in the mountains had been my main aim in coming to southern Crete. It seemed this had also been hers. It provided a point of connection with our neighbours and a good excuse to go and talk to them. Could they recommend any walks, I wondered? There were plenty of choices. Were they strenuous walks, as I had to be careful – I was convalescing. So was she, but, no, they were fine. I was recovering from chemotherapy. So was she. Trying to hide my voracious appetite for her story, on the point of leaving, but never quite making it, I asked more questions and she followed suit:

What kind of cancer have you had? (I never know which tense to use; nor she agreed, do I.)

Well, it's very rare.

So is mine.

It's called a teratoma.

A teratoma? So was mine.

You had it removed, and an ovary too?

Yes. And chemotherapy?

Bleomycin, Etopiside and Cisplatinum.

Me too.

I've got these strange scratch marks on my skin as a 'side-effect'.

So have I.

I'm having AFP tests every week.

So am I. My tests are clear so far.
So are mine. I've been taking high-dose vitamins.
So have I. I've tried all the alternative medicines.
So have I. I've been seeing a healer.
So have I. They offered me a wig, but I refused.
So did I. I've read all the cancer books.
So have I.
But I've never met anyone else ...
Nor have I.

I wanted to say, 'Tell me everything and tell me *now*. Here on the doorstep.' I could hardly bear the suspense. I was torn between a desire to stay for ever comparing all the details of our stories and my sense that we had only just met, we did not know each other and this exchange might at any moment become an intrusion. After all, we might not like each other. Having had cancer is no guarantee of friendship. And it would be hard to draw back after such confidences had been shared. But caution lost out as the pleasures of recognition drew me in. The insurmountable relief of recognition. The physical relaxation of the emotional connection. The same cancer, the same surgery, the same treatment. Some of the same side-effects. Someone else had indeed been there before, or, rather, at exactly the same time. And now, we were both here. Of all possible places, at all possible times, we had both decided to recover in this particular village on this particular week in April. More than a coincidence. A magical meeting indeed. When I got back to my flat, I wept with relief. I awoke the next day with the excitement of a six-year-old on Christmas morning.

When I returned to England and recounted this incredible narrative-of-narratives, everyone had the same response: if you put it in a novel or a film, no one would believe it. Too fictional ever to hope for, yet too coincidental to belong in good fiction. It was an encounter that defied the odds. Not only the coincidence of our meeting, but the literal coincidence of the timing of the disease and the treatment, not to mention the holiday. Our narratives told almost identical stories and we stood side by side, poised on the threshhold of recovery.

For me, this encounter is the story of my re-entry into the social world after weeks of claustrophobic internality in my physical body. There had been others around, significant others, and I had never completely lost touch with life as I had known it. But the isolation of the suffering and the impossibility of articulating its enormity had left me feeling like a stranger surrounded by familiarity. The presence of another (similar but not the same, like me but not me) enabled me to make a crucial transition out of the frozen shock of the treatment and into the world of narrative exchange. Her story made sense of mine. And my story gained substance as she listened. Unbeknownst to each of us, there had been a travelling companion on this nightmarish journey, and this offered retrospective comfort. The whole narrative could now be retold in the light of this knowledge. The similarities continued to mount as we found our common concerns extended beyond the illness to intellectual, political and cultural allegiances. I looked forward to sharing the narrative closure we both hoped for in our respective cancer stories. We would stay in touch and confirm each other's recovery as the AFP levels stayed obediently below normal.[26]

But then the pleasure of the discovery of our shared fate began to dissolve. Our paths suddenly diverged when her AFP levels went up again. We had rehearsed another story, but it escaped our control. Someone had confused the film reels again. Couldn't the power of our shared narrative pull her back towards recovery? I refused to believe that our joint physical embodiment of the survival narrative wouldn't make us immutable: surely we were now protected by the doubling effect of our encounter? But to my horror, she became the embodiment of another narrative. Our difference was cruelly underlined as her teratoma refused to be defeated. It came back again and again. More surgery and it still came back. More chemotherapy and it came back again. Surgery, intensive chemotherapy, radiotherapy. And on and on. Until finally, it had gone. Now four years later, I almost dare not say that we might both be in the clear. We still have tests. To suggest a closure at this point may tempt fate. And we haven't a shared narrative any longer. My nightmares faded into the past as hers accumulated from week to week and month to month.

The pain of separation after such blissful narrative convergence had been too much to bear. As I had gone back to work, she had gone back to hospital. As I passed my one-year threshhold, she got weaker and sicker. As I had begun to gain some distance, she had got more deeply immersed. As I had had moments of forgetting, she had had constant reminders. How to keep hoping when the stories won't oblige? What should we tell ourselves for comfort? Did she wish she were me? Did I wish she were me? If one goes down, what should the other do? These are the dangers of narrative trajectories which promise closures of certainty. What disappointments and pain they may bring instead.

VI

Cancer narratives, then, should carry a health warning: beware the certainties they promise; beware the subjects they construct; beware the truths they guarantee; and beware the closures that seem inevitable. There are variables beyond our prediction, and influences beyond our control that disrupt the easy linearity of the script. They may take us by surprise even at the moment when we feel most sure of their closure. They may change the course of the story even as the end appears to be in sight. I may have wished to write a triumph-over-tragedy story at certain moments, and some readers may want to read one (perhaps despite themselves). But I see such projects not only as disappointing to the person who does not make it, but also as potentially very worrying in terms of the cultural ideals they promise: those fantasies of omnipotence, of masculine invincibility, of individual effect.

This is not to say we should not write and rewrite the stories of our illnesses, but we should not be seduced by the power of authorship into thinking that we *alone* can determine the script. Part of my own interest in writing about my experience of cancer is to open up critical debate on precisely the fantasies around cancer which give rise to such aspirations. What is the particular appeal of these cancer narratives in contemporary culture? How do the different medical knowledges and practices which people with cancer may come across offer them particular stories about themselves and their illnesses? In order to explore these questions I have tried here and elsewhere to combine representations of my own personal narratives with a more academic account of what I think of as the changing health cultures of contemporary Western society. My motivation for writing about cancer came primarily from my experience of illness, but also from an overwhelming feeling that what was happening to me was not only horrible and terrifying, but also intellectually interesting and politically important. I found the representations of cancer intriguing from the point of view of my academic training in cultural studies and women's studies. My virtual submergence within these competing contemporary health cultures provided endless data for intellectual contemplation.

The stories of most people who suffer with cancer and other life-threatening diseases have a relatively small circulation. Few have the opportunity to have their accounts turned into print; instead their stories circulate informally, among friends, family and support groups. There are many forms of public recognition, but publication bestows status in a very particular way: it can be a form of empowerment. Academics like myself, along with other kinds of writers, have the unusual privilege to tell our stories, if we wish, and to expect others to read them and even respond to them.

My access to publishing through my academic work has enabled me to offer an account that explores some of the ways in which a person with cancer is subject to, if not bombarded with, powerful and contradictory discourses about the nature of the illness. Confusion and panic are likely responses to such a proliferation and choice of theories of cancer and how to treat it. As well as coping with the trauma and discomfort/pain of the illness, the person with cancer confronts a host of beliefs and practices which compete to define the meaning of the illness: its prevalent metaphorical manifestations, the connections between body and psyche, constructions of the healthy and the diseased self, and questions of duty and responsibility. They all offer the promise of different solutions. Some threaten recurrence if their solution is not chosen. Part of the experience of cancer in today's culture is confronting this excess of opinion about the nature of disease and the logic of the cure.

The path through the maze of information, mythology and fantasy varies according to a multitude of factors. Mine was that of an academic, highly sceptical, obsessively self-reflexive and with a sense of entitlement that feminism had added to what my class and ethnicity (middle class and white) had promised. My experience of the illness was continually inflected by the interplay of intellectual, emotional and political identifications and allegiances. At times I felt completely dependent upon medical science to save my life, while noticing (and cringing at) the heroic status I was tempted to bestow upon it. At other times I was fully engaged in alternative therapy, diets, meditation and acupuncture, accompanied by a critical analysis of their appeal. As I swallowed my vitamins every three hours, I reflected upon the profits in these renewed self-health industries (and resented my own burgeoning overdraft). As I meditated twice a day, visualizing myself cured (or even healed), I wondered about the emergent pervasiveness and persuasiveness of the healthy mind/healthy body philosophy which surrounded me.

Notes

1 The most useful of these is Trish Reynolds, *Your Cancer, Your Life* (Macdonald Optima, 1988).
2 There are hundreds of books on alternative approaches to cancer. These include books such as Penny Brohn, *Gentle Giants* and *The Bristol Programme* (both Century Publishing, 1987); Leon Chaitow *An End to Cancer* (Thorsons Publishers, 1983); Rachel Charles, *Mind, Body and Immunity* (Methuen, 1990); Michio Kushi, *The Cancer Prevention Diet* (Thorsons Publishers, 1984); O. Carl Simonton *et al.*, *Getting Well Again* (Bantam Books, 1978).

I use the term 'alternative', rather than 'complementary' or 'holistic' medicine throughout. I am aware of the debate about these terms and of the arguments about 'complementary' suggesting a more positive tone of collaboration with conventional medicine, but 'alternative' medicine is still widely used to refer to practices such as acupuncture, homoeopathy and chiropractic which are by and large still kept relatively separate from biomedical institutions and operate within an 'alternative' (and sometimes oppositional) belief system about health and healing. For a more detailed discussion of these terms, see Ursula Sharma, *Complementary Medicine Today: Practitioners and Patients* (Tavistock/Routledge, 1992).

3 See, for example, Louise Hay, *You Can Heal Your Life* and *Heal Your Body* (Eden Grove Editions, 1988; 1989) and Bernie Siegel, *Living, Loving and Healing* (Aquarian/HarperCollins, 1993). Although there is considerable overlap between this work and the kinds of books mentioned above in (2), Hay and Siegel in particular tend to be more evangelical and spiritual in tone.

4 For examples of this genre, see in particular, Brohn, *Gentle Giants*, op cit, and Charles, op cit.

5 Medical misdiagnosis is an integral part of the narrative of *Cancer in Two Voices*, a jointly written diary/memoir by Sandra Butler and Barbara Rosenblum (Spinsters Ink, 1991). Speculation about the causative effects of radiation are part of the story of her son's death from leukaemia in *Jimmy: No Time to Die* by Jane Renouf (Fontana/HarperCollins, 1993).

6 See, for example, chapter one of Nira Kfir and Maurice Slevin, *Challenging Cancer: From Chaos to Control* (Routledge, 1991) entitled 'From victims to heroes by force of circumstance'.

7 For further details on changes in the National Health System in Britain, see Ray Robinson and Julien Le Grand (eds), *Evaluating NHS Reforms* (King's Fund Institute/Policy Journals, 1994).

8 The burden of caring in the home has traditionally fallen to women, see Janet Finch and Dulcie Groves (eds), *A Labour of*

Love: Women, Work and Caring (Routledge and Kegan Paul, 1983). The cutbacks in the health service in Britain and elsewhere have doubtless increased the demands on women in this role as informal carers.

9 There is a vast critical literature on 'narrative' in English, Film and Cultural Studies. For an introduction to theories of narrative, see Shlomith Rimmon-Kenan, *Narrative Fiction and Contemporary Poetics* (Routledge, 1983).

10 For a discussion of the ways in which this basic narrative formula operates across popular film genres, see Steve Neale, *Genre* (BFI, 1980).

11 For a discussion of the place of narrative in the way we understand the 'self-identity' in late modernity see Anthony Giddens, *Modernity and Self-Identity* (Polity, 1991), especially chapter three.

12 The distinction between the public and the private in representations of the self is discussed in Derek Duncan's forthcoming study of autobiographical writing by gay men diagnosed as HIV positive. Duncan examines the autobiographies of Monette and Jarman, suggesting that 'like autobiography, AIDS insists on the public significance of private behaviour' and that 'bringing the private act of recollection into the public domain transforms a potentially solipsistic practice into an empowering political and collective challenge.' See Derek Duncan, 'Solemn Geographies: AIDS and the Contours of Autobiography' in Kate Chedgzoy and Murray Pratt (eds), *Queer Bodies* (forthcoming).

13 This refers to Duncan's title, ibid.

14 This argument is made by Duncan, who draws on Jose Arroyo's chapter 'Death, Desire and Identity: The Political Unconscious of "New Queer Cinema" ' in Joseph Bristow and Angela Wilson (eds), *Activating Theory: Lesbian, Gay and Bisexual Politics* (Lawrence and Wishart, 1993). In particular Duncan develops Arroyo's suggestion that a queer cinematic aesthetic might be characterized by 'a deep structural anxiety regarding temporality,

an anxiety ... that results from the knowledge of AIDS and its effects on the body' (Duncan, ibid). Duncan here is making a specific argument about the connections between sexual identity and health which do not parallel cancer; however, his analysis is suggestive of the ways in which illness more generally disrupts narrative coherence in relation to the projection of identities.

15 See Pete Boss's examination of how the interior of the body has become the site of horror in contemporary cinema in 'Vile Bodies and Bad Medicine', *Screen* vol 27/no 1, 1986. See also Philip Brophy, 'Horrality – the Textuality of the Contemporary Horror Film', *Screen* vol 27/no 1, 1986.

16 Boss, ibid, cites films such as *The Manitou* (1977) which deal with fears about the loss of control of the human body.

17 Sigourney Weaver stands out as a notable exception in her heroic performance in the *Alien* films. For a discussion of the gendering of cinematic heroics, see Yvonne Tasker, *Spectacular Bodies: Gender, Gore and the Action Cinema* (Routledge, 1993). The relationship between the heroine and the monster in the *Alien* films is discussed in Barbara Creed, *The Monstrous Feminine: Film, Feminism, Psychoanalysis* (Routledge, 1993).

18 See Kfir and Slevin (eds), op cit.

19 There are numerous success stories about 'conquering cancer', including Charles, op cit, Brohn, *Gentle Giants*, op cit, and Hay, *You Can Heal Your Life*, op cit.

20 Examples of media coverage of oncogene and explanation of it from *SBF.*

21 To quote this claim more fully: 'the cancer establishment ... tells you over and over again that "resistance is futile". The first radiologist I saw, a woman, called me a non-cooperator when I asked questions about the treatments and warned me that bad things would happen to me if I remained militant.' Kathleen Martindale, 'Can I Get a Witness' in *Fireweed,* no 42, 1994.

22 For a discussion of the 'defended self' in immune system discourse, see Donna Haraway, *Simians, Cyborgs and Women: The*

Reinvention of Nature (Free Association Books, 1991), chapter ten.

23 Critical analysis of 'enterprise culture' in Britain can be found in Sarah Franklin, Celia Lury and Jackie Stacey (eds), *Off-Centre: Feminism and Cultural Studies* (HarperCollins/Routledge, 1991) and Russell Keat and Nicholas Abercrombie (eds), *Enterprise Culture* (Routledge, 1991).

24 One refreshing personal account of the experience of having cancer is by Angela Wilkie, who writes about the difficulties she had with friends and family in terms of their response to her illness in *Having Cancer and How to Live With It* (Hodder and Stoughton, 1993). On a more philosophical level, Gillian Rose has written about living with cancer in her extraordinary memoir *Love's Work* (Chatto and Windus, 1995), which begins with the epitaph: 'Keep your mind in hell and despair not.'

25 Cancer support groups can be found in most towns and cities in the United Kingdom. These can be contacted through the Bristol Cancer Care Centre (01179 74321) and Back-Up (freeline 0800 181199).

26 AFP stands for alpha fetoprotein, a substance that teratoma tumours release into the blood. AFP levels thus produce a relatively reliable way of monitoring tumour activity or even cell division at a microscopic level.

Acknowledgements

Acknowledgements for a chapter about cancer could be almost as long as the chapter itself. I am hugely indebted to all those friends and family who supported me during the time of the illness, but for reasons of space, I shall only name those who have commented directly on this piece of writing. My thanks then for feedback on earlier drafts of this chapter go to Erica Carter, Claudia Casteneda, Sarah Franklin, Adrian Heathfield, Sahra Gibbon, Hilary Graham, Maureen McNeil, Lynne Pearce, Gillian Rose, Marie Shullaw, Bev Skeggs, John Urry and Mo White. In particular, I would like to thank Hilary Hinds for her generosity, patience and willingness to rehearse these critical debates at all the appropriate levels.

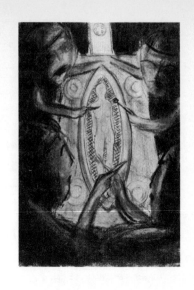

Surgery

A Remembering

Felly Nkweto Simmonds

This is not a diary but a recollection. A remembering. I began writing it in Moss, in Norway, at the end of March 1992. I had come to get away from my experience of a mastectomy in early February, and wanted to use the space between Newcastle upon Tyne and Moss to make some sense of that experience. I still write, and will probably continue to do so for as long as it takes me to make sense of my new reality.

MOSS, TUESDAY 24.3.92

I'm trying to remember too many things. I'm trying to remember what has been happening to me over the last two months as well as trying to remember a time when I was well, or rather thought I was well – apart from a chronic tooth infection and hypertension, that is.

I want to remember my body. With two breasts. With no pain. What did it feel like to have two breasts, to touch them, together or one at a time? To cradle a man's head between my naked breasts? It feels so impossible now – will I ever allow a man to see my lone (lonely) breast? I don't know if I can relate to a whole body again.

35

MOSS, WEDNESDAY 25.3.92

I have a problem with time, which is why I'm having such a problem remembering. Yet I have never been so aware of time in my life – I experience it in its absolute, with or without me, as well as in its minute form. It is nearly 2 pm and I've been up for four hours. I slept for nearly 12 hours last night. I'm in Norway for a week. In four weeks' time I go back to work. In three months' time I hope to go to Ireland. I measure it, savour it, I can almost touch it. It is tangible and also elusive. Just before I came here a friend said to me, 'I want you to come to my fortieth birthday party in Trinidad – in seven years' time.' Seven years. I can't imagine that long – I can only experience time in the present, the near future. Seven years feels like a lifetime. It could be my lifetime.

How did I relate to time BC (before cancer)? Did I feel that the future lay before me – forever? It frightens me that before the cancer was found (by chance) I thought I had time, but in fact I probably have more time to live than I had this time last year.

I kept no diary of the events I'm trying to reconstruct. I thought it would be impossible to forget. But we do forget, even pain. I had two operations. The first one, a biopsy, and then two weeks later a mastectomy. Between operations I had a horrendous infection. There were moments when I thought I'd die of blood poisoning. Now I try to remember the pain of waking up after the mastectomy – the chorus of drips, saline in my right hand, antibiotics in my left, a small sharp injection in my stomach (twice) to prevent clotting, a morphine injection in my bum for the pain, something to stop the waves of nausea rising within me. My whole body engulfed in pain, slipping in and out of consciousness, puzzled by the centre of the pain, my missing right breast. It felt as though my nipple was on fire – I could *feel* my breast, even though I knew it was in some lab, in slices, being examined. Even now, six weeks later, I can't say I feel the loss as an empty space.

MOSS, THURSDAY 26.3.92

I'm using my work diary to try to reconstruct the events of the last few months. But it is impossible to remember how I felt as I made entries such as 'cancel Govt. lecture,' 'mark dissertations,' 'interviews.' Was I scared of what might be about to happen?

It all started so casually. Sometime in November (there is *no* entry in my diary), I went for a routine cervical smear. The nurse, reading through my notes, reminds me I'm high risk for breast cancer. I'm surprised I need reminding – my mother has only been dead for two years, so why haven't I internalized the risk? Is it fear or has the feeling I've always had that it would happen to me stopped me from doing anything about it? Two years ago I watched my mother lose her life to breast cancer. It disabled me from thinking coherently about my own risk because then I would have to think about my daughter's risk, which I couldn't bear to do. How could *I*, a coward, fight the cancer which got my mother, who was so strong?

The nurse tells me that next time I come to have my blood-pressure checked, I should ask the doctor to send me for a breast screening – for my peace of mind. Looking back, I recognise that this is the moment I gained time. If she hadn't said anything, I wouldn't be here in Moss writing this. I'd be looking forward to the end of a long term at the university. I'd also be dying.

I went in for my blood-pressure check a few weeks later. It wasn't my regular doctor and I wasn't even sure whether to ask him. When I did, he told me that they might not call me in since I was only 42. But in the first post of the New Year was a letter from Newcastle General Hospital's Breast Screening Centre.

Dear Mrs Simmonds ... You may have heard that mammography is now available to women aged 40–50 years old who have a strong family history of breast cancer ...

I could have had a mammograph two years ago, but I was too busy – new job, new place, my marriage falling apart, impossible. It is odd that our bodies are the last places we visit, ignoring them at our peril, not realizing that without our bodies we have no life. We spend so much time 'sorting out' our lives, but we ignore life itself.

The appointment is for Tuesday 7 January at 11.35 am. I make a feeble attempt to get out of it by phoning to ask for another appointment, pleading pressure of work (even though I have no classes that morning), but they can't give me anything until February and I decide I can't wait that long. In the waiting room, suddenly, I realise this is no joke. There are two other women, but we avoid eye contact, each one of us in our private world of fear. I try to distract myself by looking at the magazines ... women's magazines ... BREASTS everywhere ... perfectly formed, oozing out of bras, swimsuits, dresses ... I could kill for a copy of *Marxism Today*.

Next stop, the inner waiting room. Pink plush chairs. Three changing rooms, curtained off. 'Could you just take off your top and bra, leave your cardigan on ...' Waiting. Feeling my breasts, loose and unfettered. Someone comes for me – everyone in this unit is *female*, which is a relief. The mammograph. The letter said it 'only takes a few minutes', but those minutes seem long and uncomfortable. My poor breasts squashed in the machine while the nurse escapes behind the X-ray-proof barrier. I am alone, subjected to the X-rays.

'If you don't hear from us, we'll recall you in a year.' I try to think positive, but I don't feel it. The experience has left me numb, depressed and frightened. This is the first time I've experienced the reality of being 'high risk'.

Monday 13 January, barely a week since the screening, a letter.

Dear Mrs Simmonds, Following your recent breast X-ray at the screening unit, I'd like to invite you to come to the Breast Assessment Centre ... The visit is to allow the radiographer to take more X-rays from different angles ... and, you will be examined by a doctor whilst you are there ...

INVITE! Oh shit, shit, shit, this is for *real*. The appointment is for Friday.

> About one in every ten women seen are asked to attend the second stage of screening … The majority of these women have a normal result. However, a small number of women are found to need further assessment or treatment …

Will I be one of the 'small number of women'. I've had two non-cancerous lumps removed before. I cannot be lucky third time round. I miss my mother.

There is a booklet with the letter, but I can't absorb the information. 'If you would like to bring someone with you, feel free to do so.' Who can I take?

> Eighty-five per cent of those who come to the centre will not require investigation and will be screened again in one or three years' time.

I'm not convinced, and anyway why not in two years?

> The remaining women … [What percentage is that? Fifteen? Am I one of the chosen?] … will require a breast biopsy. This involves being admitted to hospital. If this happens you will be given a date to return before you leave the Assessment Centre … Only one in three women who have a biopsy require further treatment …

I'm a statistic, but what exactly is one in three of 15 per cent? Where do *I* fit into all these statistics? And what the fuck does 'further treatment' mean? All I am told is that a biopsy 'is the removal of a small piece of tissue for examination'. I think of kleenex, which I need because I'm crying.

MOSS, FRIDAY 27.3.92

I can't imagine how I got through that week. On Friday I have to teach a two-hour seminar which starts off badly because the room has been double-booked. By the time the group re-assembles in another room, I have seriously lost the purpose of the session. After class I talk to two of the women students and try to explain why I am so distracted. They offer to come to the hospital with me, but I decline with the words 'not today, but I might need you another time'. How foolish.

Back in the now familiar waiting room I realise how badly I have underestimated the significance of this visit. There are four other women and they have *all* brought someone with them. I feel very alone – suddenly I want to cry, to hold someone's hand. Why didn't I take up the offer from my students, so concerned for me? Why do I always have to be so damned brave? I don't feel brave now. I feel ill.

I spend four hours in the Assessment Centre. I find it impossible to remember the sequence of events. X-rays … waiting for results in the pink inner waiting room. At some point one of the women (no husbands allowed here) is sobbing quietly to herself. I put my arm around her shoulders, all I can say is, 'Don't worry, it might be OK,' knowing I'm lying to her, lying to myself. She goes into the doctor's office for the final results and when she comes out, she doesn't look at me. I feel wretched. This is a bad omen.

'Mrs Simmonds …' I'm trying to absorb my new surroundings. This is the moment of truth. The doctor's office is large, bright, X-ray pictures along one wall, a large desk behind which sits a young woman doctor, a bed. The nurse who brought me in sits behind me. I want to see her face. *Listen to what the doctor is saying.* 'We have found some chalk deposits at the base of your right breast.' I feel my right nipple rise. This is not possible. The doctor is standing by the X-ray pictures, which I now realise are of my right breast. She is pointing out some white pinpoints – surely those tiny things can't be serious, they look like a fault on the film, how the hell do they even see them? 'We need to do further tests [what percentage am I now?] … A fine needle will be inserted in the area of the chalk deposits, and a blood sample will be taken ...'

Back into the screening room, my poor breast squashed again, marked, X-rayed, needle inserted, more X-rays, sample taken. The room is full of women – the Centre nurses and some district nurses on a visit, the radiographer. The cytologist, who has to take the sample, is pregnant, which comforts me. They are all so concerned, as women they know my fear. I want to cry, but I smile instead. It hurts.

MOSS, SATURDAY 28.3.92

Finally I'm called in. It is nearly 6 pm. As I walk into the doctor's office, I *know* there's something wrong. The atmosphere is different. The doctor is behind the desk, to my right. There is an empty chair to her right (was it there before?) Again, the nurse sits on a chair behind me, but I can feel her presence.

The sentence is quite simple. 'We have found some abnormal cells in the sample.' I'm sure she is saying something else, what is it? *Abnormal*. Cold, hard, it stands out from the other words in the sentence. She hesitates, waiting, and then continues, 'We have to bring you in for a biopsy ... [I've become yet another statistic] a small operation ...'

As if on cue, the door opens and a man walks in. I stare at him, knowing he is about to become *very* important to me. I observe his blue eyes, full of concern, his greying hair (I wonder how old he is). He sits on the empty chair in front of me, in his hands a large black diary, already half open. The surgeon.

He starts to explain, repeating what I have just been told. Chalk deposits, abnormal cells, biopsy, small sample for further tests – I feel as if I'm listening with a highlighter, only absorbing key words. *Thursday*.

My first words, 'Thursday is my busiest teaching day.' There is a silence. They realise that I don't seem to understand the gravity of what they are telling me. The surgeon tries again (slowly, I swear!) 'We have to do the operation as soon as possible ... I can do it this coming

Thursday … You have to take time off work.' He can see I'm not taking this in. He looks at his diary and tells me I have to come to ward 20 at 8 am next Thursday (short sentences). I take out my diary and put an entry on Thursday 23 January. 'HOSPITAL. Ward 20. Don't eat or Drink. Tea at 6 am.'

'Do you have anything you want to ask?' I sense them waiting for me to do something dramatic, cry, scream. The three of them – the doctor and surgeon in front of me, the nurse behind me – are like pillars holding me up with their concern. I can't think of a question, so I say the first thing to escape my mouth. 'I tell you what shocks me … [ah, so I *am* in shock] … it's the sheer chance of it. That the nurse at my doctor's suggested that I should start my screening because of my family history. How many women are there out there like me? It is pure chance that I am sitting here.' I'm absorbed in my thoughts, but the surgeon is talking to me, explaining my situation again. This is good, I need to hear it all again. I don't want to leave the hospital yet. Please God let me understand what this man is saying to me.

Eventually I leave the doctor's office with the breast care nurse, who takes me to her office. She gives me her card and tells me she is available at *any* time if I need her. I leave the hospital in a trance. I want to cry, but I have too much to do in the next few hours, so many phone calls to make before I leave for my weekend trip. Suddenly, a loud bang awakens me. A van and a car have collided by the hospital entrance. I hesitate for a moment, but carry on. I don't want to see blood or a mangled body. My whole body is stiff with fright. People die in car accidents in seconds. I must drive carefully tonight.

I spend the next two hours phoning friends, absorbing their shock. I try to reassure my two sons. At the airport, waiting for the plane to arrive, I'm sipping a soda water when I notice my hand is shaking. Slowly I realise that it isn't only my hand, it's my whole body shaking. The shock of the day has hit me. I put my glass down. I want to be held.

NEWCASTLE, TUESDAY 31.3.92

It is hard to remember the three days before the biopsy – teaching, a two-day workshop on Racism(!), making coherent notes in case someone has to take over, making sure all my exam questions are in. Someone phones me from a development organization in London to ask me to be a consultant on some training materials they are producing. What did I say to her? I also manage to get a message through to my husband, Paul, in Tanzania. He is coming on the first available flight and will arrive on Friday morning ... the day after the biopsy.

I'm surprised how well I sleep on Wednesday night, to be awakened by my radio alarm at 5.30 am. I have a long bath, I caress my breasts, paying special attention to my right breast, still bruised from the needle test. I need a man to touch this breast, but I'm alone. This was the last full bath I would have for over a month.

My friend, Mave, arrives at 8 am to take me to hospital. My sons are coming with me – I want them to feel part of what is going on. I think of my daughter, away at university; I'm relieved she is not here to witness this. Hospital reception, filling in forms, up to ward 20. Mave and the boys stay as long as possible, which isn't very long. When they leave I feel utterly alone.

I don't want to be in hospital. I'm fine. What am I doing here with all these sick people?

Hours of pre-operation routine. They come for me after lunch (what lunch?) Somehow I get on to the trolley without exposing my bum. Down the corridor, into the lift, down another corridor. Everyone from now on is in green. They smile reassuringly. More questions – name, date of birth, address, do you know what the operation entails? I've been asked the same questions at least five times during the morning. The anaesthetist. I know my life will be in his hands. He is Asian, Kenyan Asian; I decide I'll be OK. I like him. The anaesthetist is talking to me. I try to say something in Kiswahili, but can't remember a word. He's patting the back of my left hand and I try not to watch as I feel the needle go into my vein.

I feel odd. Someone is calling my name, asking me how I feel. I'm completely awake. A male nurse is sitting by my bed, talking to me, trying to make me say something. All I can say is 'it hurts'.

My right breast is a lump of pain, all bandaged up. There's a tube coming out of the bandage. I hurt. I feel sick. All I want to do is sleep. I feel myself being wheeled back to the ward. The movement makes my nausea worse. I'm asleep as soon as they put me back in my bed … for hours, until I'm woken by the sickness. I manage to attract the attention of a nurse who, just in time, hands me a small bowl into which I'm sick. I'm in such pain I don't know what to do with myself. The ward sister offers me morphine for the pain and something for the sickness. At this point even injections are bliss … and sleep.

Early evening, Mave and the boys come to see me, laden with flowers, fresh orange juice, water, sweets. The orange juice tastes like nectar, or what I think nectar might taste like. I try to talk and smile, but have no idea whether I'm succeeding.

It is not until the following morning that I begin to absorb my surroundings. I feel out of place, everyone else is white. Sometime in the morning I catch a glimpse of an Asian woman in the next ward. The previous day I had tried not to watch the other women on the ward, but now I'm fascinated by the various attachments they carry with them – drips, oxygen and either a single tube or two coming out from their nightdresses into little paper bags that they carry with them as they visit each other's beds to compare flowers, cards, share sweets. They all looked quite cheerful and I wondered what they were in for. Now it all falls into place – I too have a single tube from my bandaged breast, draining into a bottle by my bed. Later I too am given a small paper carrier bag to put my bottle in, advertising some perfume. On the bag is a most startling image: Elizabeth Taylor in a swimming pool, looking coy, two perfectly formed breasts oozing out of her costume. I feel sick – is this some cruel joke, giving us these bags at a time when we couldn't be more conscious of other women's apparently healthy breasts?

I stayed in ward 20 for just one night, no time even to get on nodding terms with the other women. On Friday many go home; I and the few remaining are moved to ward 19. I can't be bothered to adjust to the new faces, so I keep my head low and try not to think about my throbbing breast. They let me out on the third day after my operation – one of the effects of the lack of funding of the National Health Service is that hospitals can't keep patients in for longer than absolutely necessary, there are always others waiting for beds. The cost of such rationalization is human, and I paid for it in the following week.

Going home is wonderful, the house full of flowers and cards, phone call after phone call from my friends. I don't think I've ever felt so loved. But there is an underlying certainty that every so often catches up with me, leaving me in tears. I cannot predict what will set it off. First, there is the idea of waiting for the results ... for five days. How will these days pass?

By Sunday evening I know there is an infection. My breast has swollen to twice its normal size and I'm in agony. I also have a temperature. When my GP arrives he is visibly shocked by the state of my breast, and prescribes antibiotics. By Wednesday night we have to call the emergency doctor followed by an ambulance ride to casualty. Over my head the word operation is mentioned. Back in ward 19 I get another red 'nil by mouth' sign. This is pure hell. The surgeon on call comes and removes nearly 100 ml of 'dead blood'. The relief is immediate. I also get an intravenous drip for antibiotics, burning all the way up my vein, and saline to wash the burning sensation. I ache in every bit of my body – I now cannot remember what it feels like to have no pain. I'm also so thirsty.

The morning round brings my surgeon who reassures me and asks a nurse to give me a cup of tea. No operation. All I have to do now is wait for my results ... after lunch on Friday.

On Friday I fret all morning, unable to sleep. Just as lunch is being served in the next ward I fall into a deep sleep, oblivion. I miss lunch and the surgeon's visit. He doesn't have the heart to wake me up. When I do wake it is nearly visiting time and soon Paul arrives. For nearly two hours we talk and wait. I fret, watching the door. By 5.30 I can't wait any longer and ask Paul to ask the nurse when the surgeon will come.

Almost casually she tells me he has been, while I was asleep. I'll get the results the next morning. It is hard to believe that she is saying this to me ... hot tears run down my face. 'You people have no idea what this waiting is like ... I'm going home ... I will not stay in this hospital tonight.' Between sobs I manage to say this, without swearing, which is all I want to do. The nurse disappears. I hang on to Paul's hand, sobbing loudly. There's a hush in the ward – apparently tears are embarrassing. 'Fuck them,' I think.

After what seems like a fraction of a minute the nurse reappears with the surgeon. I can't stop crying as he asks me what is upsetting me. At some point the curtains are drawn around my bed – to protect me, or the rest of the ward from my tears? The surgeon perches on the arm of the chair beside my bed. His hands are tight fists on my bed as he leans forward. His knuckles are white. He looks tired.

'I can tell you the results now ... we have found that there is a cancer in your right breast ...'

I feel so light. Have I stopped breathing? Why is it so silent? All I can hear is his voice, as if in a vacuum. I swear there's no other sound in the world except this man's voice.

'... a cancer in your right breast ...' Did he say it twice or did I hear it twice? As he says it I feel my right breast detach itself from the rest of my body. It is no longer part of me. It has a cancer. I don't have cancer.

'... It is in its early stages ... A ductal carcinoma in situ ... still contained in the ducts ... has not invaded the breast tissue or the lymph nodes ... but the whole breast tissue is unstable ... a slow-growing cancer, you've probably had it two or three years ...'

My mother – that's when I got it. The moment my mother died. Will I ever forget the moment I looked at my mother's face, so peaceful, she'd only been dead a few minutes. I'd missed her by minutes. Watching myself on the floor beside the bed, disintegrating, howling, what is that noise, surely it can't be me? Being carried out of the ward by my brother as my father talks to my mother, touching her face.

'My recommendation is that I remove the breast, thus ensuring that the whole cancer is removed ...'

My eyes are tightly shut. All I can see is red. Through the redness I hear his voice, quiet, concerned. I'm crying, thinking of my beautiful 18-year-old daughter. How can I leave her such a legacy? My first question. 'How much danger is my daughter in?' 'Yes, she is at risk, and we have to keep an eye on her from when she is 30.' But he wants me to think about myself at this moment.

So many things are explained. At various points the surgeon waits for me to say something, but I can't. He tells me the nature of the cancer, the options available, his recommendation, the mastectomy, the post-mastectomy treatment, Tamoxifen, breast reconstruction. He gives me all this information slowly, clearly. I'm surprised that I do understand, everything, perfectly. I've already made my decision. I want the breast off. The surgeon wants me to think about it, but I tell him I don't need to wait. I'd lived with this possibility for seven years. It is all quite clear to me and I feel quite calm, except for a burning sensation in the centre of my chest and the tears I'm struggling to control. The surgeon thinks I'm being too calm and sends me home with the words 'Go home and have a good cry …' What a wise man!

Before I leave I'm given the date of the mastectomy, 10 February 1992, 16 days before my forty-third birthday.

POSTSCRIPT, NOVEMBER 1994

It is over two and a half years since I wrote 'A Remembering'. In the meantime I have moved on. Physically I'm in better health than at any time I can remember; psychologically I've had to climb mountains to reach a level where I feel at peace with myself; emotionally the experience of a mastectomy has forced me to change not only how I relate to myself, but also to other people. The further I get from the experience, the more I realise what an impact it has had on my life. It seems that losing a breast has allowed me to 'lose' other things and people I thought I couldn't live without. I have learned to live with these losses; each day I get better at managing loss and feel better for it.

A close friend who read 'A Remembering' a year after I wrote it commented on the omissions and lack of anger. As far as the omissions are concerned, there were many traumatic things going on which linked into my experience of cancer, but which I can't include in a public re-telling of that experience. Some things will remain mine alone, some I share with the women closest to me or with my children. I still haven't found a positive way of sharing this experience with men – perhaps this will come when I'm more secure in myself, in my body. In time I may be able to talk about how various bits of my world collided, leaving me fragmented.

I remember two days after the operation looking at my body for the first time in a full-length mirror with utter disbelief. The face I could place, but nothing else. Knowing there and then I'd never let a man see this body. Feeling *nothing*. I didn't know what I should feel.

The anger came much later, when I could feel something. At first the sheer pain of the operations reduced me to a level of self-pity I don't think I could survive again. I was suicidal for most of May and all of August. In September I found myself getting seriously angry, but by then I couldn't share this anger with many people – it seemed unfair to keep on dragging my friends down with me. I still get angry now. I don't want to be one-breasted.

The moment I began to get angry at the unfairness of it all was when I went to see the London Contemporary Dance group at the Newcastle Theatre Royal, my first outing on my own since the mastectomy. In the audience was one of the junior doctors from the hospital – *he* knew I had only one breast, that I was different from the other women, from the woman he was with. For the first time I felt disabled; I wondered how people in wheelchairs can bear to see others walk. Sitting alone among all the healthy white couples, death seemed preferable.

The performance, by contrast, was wonderfully alive. I found myself mesmerised by the young women's bodies, especially the black women, so healthy, so young. For a long time after my mastectomy all I could see of women was the shape of their breasts. Is this how men see women? I became so obsessed that when I met a woman for the first time, I'd remember the shape of her chest – no face, no name. It was pure madness. Of course, the irony is that since I wear a prosthesis I look the same as everybody else. I would like to be able to wear a badge that says 'I'm one-breasted,' but I'm not so brave.

That evening plummeted me into a deep depression – I felt I would never get used to it, didn't want to get used to it, wanted to die. I cried from 2 am til 4 am, took a sleeping pill which worked only until 7.30 am, and at 10 am, completely out of my head, phoned my friend Uma. She came to talk to me. I told her I wanted to die but she wouldn't let me.

That first year I rediscovered the power of tears. Whenever I felt I might lose control I would go home by the quickest possible route and *cry*. I used to cry in short, sharp bursts, to clear the head, before I went to work; or when I was desperate to be held, to be reassured, I would take myself to bed and cry. I also experienced long 'healing' sleeps, sometimes 12 hours at a stretch, with dreams of being alone and happy or of being one-breasted. This made my body feel less alien, made me feel I might get used to it.

Now I have become a new woman, in ways that surprise me. I have had to learn to love myself in a way I never did when I thought I was well, when the idea of dying wasn't part of my living. I'm less anxious about life, I live each day experiencing the emotions the day brings, be they joyful or painful. I try to heal each hurt as I experience it, and not to ignore it, so I don't carry too many anxieties in my body. It's hard work, but I feel that in the long run it pays off.

I was brought up a 'good Catholic girl' and my life had become one of giving, to everyone except myself. Sometimes when I play *Beatitudes*, by Sweet Honey in The Rock, I remember the philosophy I was taught:

> Blessed are the Meek for they shall inherit the Earth.
> Blessed are the Merciful, for they shall obtain Mercy.
> Blessed are the Peacemakers, for they shall be called the Children of God ...

Though I haven't been a practising Catholic for half my life, the funda-mental stuff was still there. Looking back, I'm amazed at the things I tolerated, my carelessness about my own needs. I think this contributed to my ill health – I had learned to bottle up emotions, especially anger.

Anger was one of the first things I had to learn to deal with. I was angry because I had spent my life being a good woman, a good mother, a good wife, and my 'blessing' was the loss of a breast. First I learned to feel this anger, which would leave me exhausted for days on end, and then I learned to express anger in words. Now when people hurt me I ring them up and tell them, I write letters. I refuse to carry the pain and anger of feeling taken for granted – I allow myself not only to experience anger but to confront the cause, however risky and painful. As a result I have lost several people I was close to.

I have lost some friends and lovers. My marriage has ended. But in a way these losses free me from burdens I'm no longer willing to carry.

The mastectomy changed my relationship to myself and to other people. At first the trauma of the experience made me retreat into an angry inner self from which I emerged only gradually. I have become more self-focused, some may call it selfish. I'm much clearer about what I can ask of people and what can be asked of me. As a result have also made new and unexpected friendships that give me a new sense of self, a new place of safety. I allow myself to be loved for what I am, not for what I can provide. This has given me the most unexpected joy.

At the heart of this change is my relationship with death. I'm no longer afraid to die, but I want to live before I die. In the past two years one of my brothers and a close male friend have died. Their deaths left me very angry, especially since they were both younger than me. It makes me even more determined to live in the here and now and not focus on what could be. Now I *choose* what and whom I spend my energies on and focus on those things and people that sustain me. I nurture friendships which give me energy and life, and detach myself from those which don't. I nurture without allowing myself to be exploited.

I look after myself physically, going to the gym twice a week not only to get fit but to get in touch with my body. To feel my body and to be alone with myself. I have learned to listen to my body and know when enough is enough. I regularly spend a Saturday or Sunday in bed, reading, writing, watching TV and pampering myself.

I look after myself emotionally. I'm much more honest about admitting what I feel and acting on it. I also allow myself to enjoy emotions and relationships that until recently I would have judged 'unsuitable'. I enjoy relationships being loved for what they are at the time, not for what they could be in some future I might not have.

I write to get in touch with what I'm experiencing. I have learned through therapy to have one place where I have to be completely honest, and that is my diary. I do not write every day, but regularly enough to work out tensions and make sense of particular experiences. I know when I'm hiding something from myself, or trying to avoid something, by the gaps in my diary. My diary is the place I get in touch with my spirit, recounting events and dreams. If I ever have a grand-daughter, I would like to leave her my diaries and my 'spirit' name – Nkweto wa Chilinda – in the hope that she may work out what my life was about when I finally took control of it.

I have also learned to be alone. I no longer have a live-in partner, and my children, now grown up, no longer live at home. For the first time in my life I have my own space, space where I can just be. Sometimes, like now, I love the silence of the night which I use to think, to read and to write. Most times I listen to music – Baaba Maal, Ella Fitzgerald, Billie Holiday; a drop of whisky beside me.

I have learned to value the people who see me through the bad times I still have, those who recognize and accept my weaknesses, even my selfishness at times – my friends, old and new, and my children: Clare Nkweto, Peter Mumbi and Tom Chewe, who have given me the space to learn that I don't always have to be a 'good mother'. *Asante sana watoto wangu.*

For the first time in my life, I feel at peace with myself.

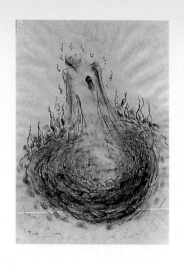

Radiotherapy

Cancer Winter

Marilyn Hacker

For Rafael Campo and Hayden Carruth

Syllables shaped around the darkening day's
contours. Next to armchairs, on desks, lamps
were switched on. Tires hissed softly on the damp
tar. In my room, a flute concerto played.
Slate roofs glistened in the rain's thin glaze.
I peered out from a cave like a warm bear.
Hall lights flicked on as someone climbed the stairs
across the street, blinked out: a key, a phrase
turned in a lock, and something flew open.
I watched a young man at his window write
at a plank table, one pooled halogen
light on his book, dim shelves behind him, night
falling fraternal on the flux between
the odd and even numbers of the street.

                    *   *   *

I woke up, and the surgeon said, 'You're cured.'
Strapped to the gurney, in the cotton gown
and pants I was wearing when they slid me down

onto the table, made new straps secure
while I stared at the hydra-headed O.R.
lamp, I took in the tall, confident, brown-
skinned man, and the ache I couldn't quite call pain
from where my right breast wasn't anymore
to my armpit. A not-yet-talking head,
I bit dry lips. What else could he have said?
And then my love was there in a hospital coat;
then my old love, still young and very scared.
Then I, alone, graphed clock-hands' asymptote
to noon, when I would be wheeled back upstairs.

* * *

The odd and even numbers of the street
I live on are four thousand miles away
from an Ohio February day
snow-blanketed, roads iced over, with sleet
expected later, where I'm incomplete
as my abbrievated chest. I weigh
less – one breast less – since the Paris-gray
December evening, when a neighbor's feet
coming up ancient stairs, the feet I counted
on paper were the company I craved.
My calm right breast seethed with a grasping tumor.
The certainty of my returns amounted
to nothing. After terror, being brave
became another form of gallows humor.

* * *

At noon, an orderly wheeled me upstairs
via an elevator hung with Season's
Greetings streamers, bright and false as treason.
The single room the surgeon let us share
the night before the knife was scrubbed and bare
except for blush-pink roses in a vase on
the dresser. Veering through a morphine haze on

the cranked bed, I was avidly aware
of my own breathing, my thirst, that it was over –
the week that ended on this New Year's Eve.
A known hand held, while I sipped, icewater,
afloat between ache, sleep, lover and lover.
The one who stayed would stay; the one would leave.
The hand that held the cup next was my daughter's.

          *   *   *

It's become a form of gallows humor
to reread the elegies I wrote
at that pine table, with their undernote
of cancer as death's leitmotiv, enumer-
ating my dead, the unknown dead, the rumor
of random and pandemic deaths. I thought
I was a witness, a survivor, caught
in a maelstrom and brought forth, who knew more
of pain than some, but learned it loving others.
I need to find another metaphor
while I eat up stories of people's mothers
who had mastectomies. 'She's eighty-four
this year, and *fine!*' Cell-shocked, I brace to do
what I can, an unimportant exiled Jew.

          *   *   *

The hand that held the cup next was my daughter's
– who would be holding shirts for me to wear,
sleeve out, for my bum arm. She'd wash my hair
(not falling yet), strew teenager's disorder
in the kitchen, help me out of the bathwater.
A dozen times, she looked at the long scar
studded with staples, where I'd suckled her,
and didn't turn. She took me/I brought her
to the surgeon's office, where she'd hold
my hand, while his sure hand, with its neat tool, snipped
the steel, as on a revised manuscript

radically rewritten since my star
turn nursing her without a 'nursing bra'
from small, firm breasts, a twenty-five-year-old's.

*   *   *

I'm still alive, an unimportant Jew
who lives in exile, voluntarily
or not: Ohio's alien to me.
Death follows me home here, but I pay dues
to stay alive. White cell count under two:
a week's delay in chemotherapy
stretches it out. Ohio till July?
The Nazarenes and Pentecostals who
think drinking wine's a mortal sin would pray
for me to heal, find Jesus, go straight, leave.
But I'm alive, and can believe I'll stay
alive a while. Insomniac with terror
I tell myself, it isn't the worst horror.
It's not Auschwitz. It's not the Vel d'Hiv.

*   *   *

I had 'breasts like a twenty-five-year-old,'
and that was why, although a mammogram
was done the day of my year-end exam
in which the doctor found the lump, it told
her nothing: small, firm, dense breasts have and hold
their dirty secrets till their secrets damn
them. Out of the operating room
the tumor was delivered, sanctioned, cold-
packed, pickled, to demonstrate to residents
an infiltrative ductal carcinoma
(with others of its kind). I've one small, dense
firm breast left, and cell-killer pills so no more
killer cells grow, no eggs drop. To survive
my body stops dreaming it's twenty-five.

56

It's not Auschwitz. It's not the Vel d'Hiv.
It's not gang-rape in Bosnia or
gang-rape and gutting in El Salvador.
My self-betraying body needs to grieve
at how hatreds metastasize. Reprieved
(if I am), what am I living for?
Cancer, gratuitous as a massacre,
answers to nothing, tempts me to retrieve
the white-eyed panic in the mortal night,
my father's silent death at forty-eight,
each numbered, shaved, emaciated Jew
I might have been. They wore the blunt tattoo,
a scar, if they survived, oceans away.
Should I tattoo my scar? What would it say?

* * *

No body stops dreaming it's twenty-five
or twelve, or ten, when what is possible's
a long road poplars curtain against loss, able
to swim the river, hike the culvert, drive
through the open portal, find the gold hive
dripping with liquid sweetness. Risible
fantasy, if, all the while, invisible
entropies block the roads, so you arrive
outside a ruin, where trees bald with blight
wane by a river drained to sluggish mud.
The hovering swarm has nothing to forgive.
The setting sun looks terribly like blood.
Your querulous voice whines to indifferent night:
'I don't know how to die yet. Let me live.'

* * *

Should I tattoo my scar? What would it say?
It could say 'K.J.'s Truck Stop' in plain English, highlighted with a nipple ring
(the French version: Chez KJ/Les Routiers).

I won't be wearing falsies, and one day
I'll bake my chest again at Juan-les-Pins,
round side and flat, gynandre/androgyne,
close by my love's warm flanks (though she's sun-shy
as I should be: it's a carcinogen
like smoked fish, caffeine, butterfat and wine).
O let me have my life and live it too!
She kissed my breasts, and now one breast she kissed
is dead meat, with its pickled blight on view.
She'll kiss the scar, and then the living breast.

*   *   *

I don't know how to die yet. Let me live!
Did Etty Hillesum think that, or Anne Frank,
or the forty-year-old schoolteacher the bank
robber took hostage when the cop guns swiv-
eled on them both, or the seropositive
nurse's aide who, one long-gone payday, drank
too much, fucked whom? or the bag lady who stank
more than I wished as I came closer to give
my meager change? I say it, bargaining
with the *contras* in my blood, immune
system bombarded but on guard. Who's gone?
The bookseller who died at thirty-nine,
poet, at fifty-eight, friend, fifty-one,
friend, fifty-five. These numbers do not sing.

*   *   *

She'll kiss the scar, and then the living breast,
and then, again, from ribs to pit, the scar,
but only after I've flown back to her
out of the unforgiving Middle West
where my life's strange, and flat disinterest
greets strangers. At Les Saintes-Maries-de-la-Mer,
lust pulsed between us, pulsed in the plum-grove where
figs dropped to us like manna to the blessed.

O blight that ate my breast like worms in fruit,
be banished by the daily pesticide
that I ingest. Let me live to praise
her breathing body in my arms, our wide-
branched perennial love, from whose taproot
syllables shape around the lengthening days.

*   *   *

Friends, you died young. These numbers do not sing
your requiems, your elegies, our war
cry: at last, not 'Why me?' but 'No more
one-in-nine, one-in-three, rogue cells killing
women.' You're my companions, travelling
from work to home to the home I left for
work, and the plague, and the poison which might cure.
The late sunlight, the morning rain, will bring
me back to where I started, whole, alone,
with fragrant coffee into which I've poured
steamed milk, book open on the scarred pine table.
I almost forgot how close to the bone
my chest's right side is. Unremarkable,
I woke up, still alive. Does that mean 'cured'?

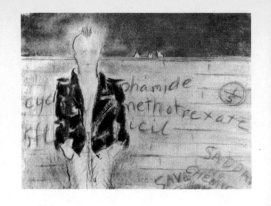

Chemotherapy

Sweat

Jacqueline Julien

For Denise, murdered

Truth is a fire that burns whatever is false. Truth is a hard but hardwearing cushion on which we sit after having danced too long in circles. When our thoughts stray from the path of truth, sometimes what they reveal is simply the other side of cloth they have wearied of weaving.

Christine Boomester, painter

OPEN WOUND I

You are sweating. It is a sign. You have started to sweat. Your body and the air, as one, return this sticky water to you. Blindly, you stare at the sheath that clings to your skin. You don't believe in the evil spell of the heat of the air. Many other kinds of heat have run softly over this body or your body has produced sweat from its own heat – this murky moisture that made your skin shine. Her body was whispering against yours, sliding smoothly against this sheath that your whispering skins crushed. Caught up in the art of pleasure, you were deaf to the whisper of your skins. You liked the sweat of your two bodies, the combination of wetnesses, her hair running down her neck, soaked. Everything wet, from her body on to yours.

You have been calling yourself 'you' since her death. You have begun to refer to yourself as 'you'. But this 'you' is not the you of the living. You remember that after the war those survivors who had lost everything, to the point of belonging nowhere that bore a name, were classified as 'Displaced Persons'. This 'you' you have substituted for your ruined 'I', for yourself, defiled by the loss of everything, is the *you* of a displaced person. The 'you' you used to call her was offered as a gift, echoing with everything that defined the two of you together, alive. Her death has stolen that 'you'. Her death has swept away any possible 'I'.

You are placed on the sheet. You are sweating. The sweat melts you, erases you, blurs your outline. You do not recognise your belly, your knees, your thighs. You know nothing of your neck, your pores, your hair. It is no longer your hair. All you know is that this sweat is the hideous mistress of your pain. You have no other choice but pain. Pain and sweat mean the same thing; it has nothing to do with the heat of the afternoon. Other kinds of heat have run softly over your body; other heats have set your skin on fire; other positions on this sheet have sheathed your skin with a different sweat from this sweat now, on your motionless body.

The sheet is a shroud in waiting. No, not yet. A shroud would be fresh and crisp, newly unfolded. This sheet stewed in your sweat, your wet disorder, cannot be a shroud. You recall other times when you have lain in this bed, other afternoons – those little nights of day. Or rather they enter your mind unbidden, jumbled like unfiled letters. You have become accustomed to this jumble of someone who is dying. A little film skipping on the fragments of your involuntary memories.

Another time, yes, you had been very ill, as one can only be when one is in good health. A nasty bronchitis that taught you to like vegetable stock. Her hand held out the bowl. There was a smile in her hand as it stroked your forehead, waited for the empty bowl you returned to her, cracked open the capsules, brought the syrup to your lips. What did it matter that you were ill? It was winter, it was an excuse to go to bed early together, the bed that smelled of her perfume, your fever, suppository. That made you both laugh, that childhood smell.

You held happiness.

Other afternoons, probably in summer or perhaps in May: a drought, a dust, a certain amount of crickets or a premature stubble clearing that made it feel like summer. The doors and windows are open to the confused bees that come crashing into the walls. You are walking together barefoot in the house. You ask her to hang out the washing. Later on it is you who folds it. The cat follows you, happily. You hear without listening your neighbour nailing something together, you are waiting for the grocery van – the sound of its horn like a cheerful pollutant. Depending, you sometimes do and sometimes don't join the elderly women who slowly gather round the temporary stall. You are not always in the mood to greet them individually or to discuss today's wind or the wind that is surely on its way. You really have to have run out of salt or butter. Sometimes it is making love together that prevents you from getting there in time.

The rule in the village is that the weather is a cause for complaint rather than for celebration. You can guess at the reasons for this ritual of collective suspicion, but sometimes you are just too happy. You would be incapable of lying in order to join in with the chorus of the elderly women who dread nice weather because of the storm that will surely follow, who dread happiness because of the misfortune it heralds. You were holding happiness and nothing could induce you to let it go. Neither of you knew anything of misfortune.

The window, to your left, is a white hole. You stare diligently at the white hole of the window. Then you turn your eyes to the wall facing the bed and bore the white hole of the window into the wall. Piercing the wall with the white hole of the window is your occupation. You are very ill. There isn't any syrup to take. There is no longer that childhood smell in the bed that made you both laugh. There is this coma, though. There is that you are dying, bathed in sweat.

You have been left for alive, but it was a mistake. Your life and her death are incompatible. There is no way that you could be in two places at the same time, which is what it would require. There is no possible accord between her death, where you are not, and life, which has held on to you. You quickly understood that it would not be possible. There was no room in your life for her death.

You stare with your blind eyes at the blind hole in the wall. You are sweating. Other windows open wide like an abyss. You are not doing it deliberately. They just open. To the confused bees that come crashing into the walls, which you would both sweep out with a tea towel. To the hammering from your neighbour who is always nailing something together and does not greet either of you anymore since he heard your cries.

The windows open onto the cleared stubble crowned with sunflowers. To the cat that returns from its inspection of the hen house. To the washing which was waiting to be taken down before the rain, but too late, the rain has arrived and neither of you did anything but hear it from the bedroom. To the sound of the horn that covers your sighs. To the close-up of her face that fills the frame.

Together you held happiness.

The putrid smell of your sweat rises from the sticky sheet. It floats upwards, filling the lower half of the room, then expands further, impregnating the whole space laid open to it. You recognise this smell of decay. Her death taught you the smell of carrion, that last flowering of her life that penetrated your skin until it in turn exuded the juice of its final agony. Smelling on you that smell of her death brings you closer to her death. More precisely, her death visits you. You feel more alive, having smelled her death as well as your own. Death, the smell of death, you have to be so fully alive to recognise it. Animals are aware of it first. The cat had recognised it. The cat was keeping its distance, sick at not being able to do anything more.

It never purred again.

There was the afternoon of the smell which is the climax of all smells, we learned that. The dominant one. Shit follows: the funeral procession. Shit is just the maid of agony. And far behind, over-whelmed, is the greater smell of love. But it was greater, you both held it for greater. The smell of love, the mistress of your awakening and your sleeping. At the time you did not know the dominant smell. So you held the smell of love to be the greatest – all other smells, whether delightful fragrances or unpleasant stenches you encountered on your journeys together (among which a memorable Paris-Milan train ride where you were unable to sleep because of the smell of body odour in the compartment) were minor in comparison. However foul or exhilarating this or that was pronounced, none of them would ever have been ranked with that greatest of mysteries, the smell of love. You held the smell. You didn't yet know the dominant one.

There was the afternoon when you smelled it for the first time. Perhaps it wasn't the first time, but it was the first time you understood what it was. You tried to believe it was something else: a dead field-mouse the cat had abandoned, carrion in the ditch by the road (the window was open, it was a hot day, you never know). But this was it, the dominant one, it had come. In the evening, stretched out on the narrow divan you had placed beside her bed, you had sniffed the smell of her death on your hands, under your nails. No soap could rid you of it, no eau-de-Cologne, no sleep.

The cat had cleared off.

There was the afternoon before her coma. For days now the house had been home to the dominant smell: its strength depends not only on the law of volumes, but on the structure of the house, the thickness of the walls, the cracks between the floorboards. As soon as you entered the house you breathed it in, despite yourself. In the cool hallway it faded into an illusion as your steps distanced you from the epicentre on the first floor; or your nostrils, on the defensive, would temporarily anaesthetise you to the stench revealed as you entered. The kitchen was further away from the epicentre by foot, but a smell does not travel in terms of steps. It spreads like an invisible hailstorm, as the ghost flies, it slips through the cracks between the floorboards, showers you with its gas.

The kitchen, located below the epicentre, implodes. You are defeated and every step you take towards the first floor is a step towards abomination. At the door there is no longer any distance between yourself and the smell. You are the smell. It is no longer simply a smell, it is a flavour that wets your lips, your tongue, your teeth.

Later, at the hospital, the nurses were weeping, exhausted. The entire ward had been taken over by the rot that triggered your senses from the ground floor. They were saying that the patients were terrified and wouldn't stop complaining.

There was the afternoon of her coma. You are watching her death, which abandons you to your life. But she doesn't understand this desertion. There is no final message, no awareness of a farewell, of a necessary parting. Since the arrival of the dominant smell you are the only one to have recognised what is happening. You have not been able to share it with her.

Her arms have been rowing thin air.

There was the afternoon of her absence, you have not said of her death. No, that can't be said straight away. Probably because you have been aware of it for some time, not as the death of another but as a death descended from yourself. Before her death, there was her desertion. Her absence in your life began with your absence in hers. You have been left for alive, but it was a mistake. You have been abandoned to your life. The rediscovery of the smell of her death on you, this visitation, comforts you slightly.

All is not lost.

Marginal Notes: June

I am uncovering in real time the mechanism that is forcing me to come to terms with her death and with my death from her death, to introduce myself in this way, as a voyeur of dreams and of agony. So it will be uncovered for you at the same time as it is uncovered for me. I acknowledge that the story to be unfolded must seem monstrous to you, a dreadful mystification. But I sense also that this necessarily mystificatory narration will also be enlightening and salutary.

You have to be so alive to write about death, so incredibly alive, just like cancer. My cancer, which writes about the death in the body of my life, is a model of vitality. As a writer I like to take it as a model. It enables me to recover the ferocious, massive energy of which I have long been deprived, or of which I have deprived myself, for obscure reasons which I will of necessity discover. I can see the same concentration as well as this metaphor of secrecy that is so appropriate to my life as a writer. What I write remains secret as long as the hidden (one might say lethal) meaning is well woven into it, and until an additional but uncontrollable impulse tears off the lid to reveal (one might say bring to life) death : the unknown element that was being created within it.

And so cancer, my contracted and concealed cancer, has developed its own language, an anti-language, a nocturnal writing before its exposure, before the publication of the banns of its genesis.

Here the writing, my writing, is exposed.

Here the tumour that gave birth to the work of darkness is exposed. So clear after having lived in shadow, flesh of my flesh, both womb and mother, language and speech, humus and forest. Here is the undesired monster, exposed. Abandoned to the next salutary ferocity.

Born from the condensation of confessed deliriums and unconfessable confessions, these cells that play by the rules of another game – revolutionary, lethal, tempting – re-open a closed channel.

These marginal notes are the towpath.

OPEN WOUND II

The white hole of the window has become a greyish screen.

The wall opposite the bed can't be bored any further. You let your head lean towards the bleak rectangle that frames the twilight. The wind is rising, you listen to the wind creeping around the house, climbing like a vine. The nurse will soon arrive with her 'It's me!' full of controlled enthusiasm. It's the same nurse, the same sleek young lady, impervious to rot, disinfected, never late. Cleansing and dressing with the unctuous hands of a pastry chef, injecting while chattering and setting off again without feeling any remorse.

Then comes the night nurse, whose arrival you dread because you so hate the night.

She has closed the window, switched on the lamp. You shiver in the fresh, dry sheets, stretched too tightly. You feebly move your feet in an effort to release yourself, incapable of turning over, tortured by the desire to do so, condemned to the pain of your crushed coccyx, your imprisoned spine. You dream of your bodies making love, your baby postures. Your belly dreams of the weight of your body lying face down, the weight of her body face down on yours. You have nothing to dream about. You're in waiting. Your pain waits with you for its morphine hood.

Tomorrow the ambulance will take you back to hospital. That will make life easier for your friends. Their healthy faces leaning over you will intercept the chrome pipes, the white lacquered arches. The smells of the city they bring will be defeated at the doorway. You will be sleeping: your friends will be disappointed but relieved. You will be sleeping more and more often, but only you will know that you're not sleeping, only your pain is sleeping in its morphine hood. Your friends will leave you a note of regret on a cheerful card. You will bore holes in the wall opposite the bed. You will feebly move your feet to release yourself from the sweaty sheets, again stretched too tightly. You will try to remember the wind that surrounded the house at twilight, creeping like an animal wanting to get in.

This may be the last evening you'll watch the twilight arrive in the bleak rectangle of the window, that you'll hear the wind. Hospital is much more convenient for agony, for friends who want to come and visit you after work. Wind can't be heard in hospital, perhaps this is the last time you'll hear the wind creeping around the house.

The morphine has filled your blood, colonised your veins, your arteries, your nerves.

Your pain is melting away into its strait-jacket, laced tight by your heartbeats.

The chariot that brings your sleepless dreams is arriving.

Kàrola, pronounced with a stress on the *kà*, tonight Kàrola spares you the oblivion that has cracked open your memory like an axe-blow. On the butcher's block where separation smashed you to pieces, your brain spilled out its contents and your memories, forever fractured, ran into the sawdust. Often, gathering up the stressed *kà* of Kàrola, hoping to put together the lost name with the beloved face, you would trip on the other face, as if some badly connected circuits had diverted the answer to your command. Communication failure, cut off at so many levels, both elementary – her name, her face – and vital, has instigated this automatic withdrawal of your memory, placed it in an involuntary sphere where remembering and forgetting both starve and feed each other. You hardly dared risk gathering up the *kà* of Kàrola. It was no longer automatic to say *Kàrola*, to see her, to feel her warmth, this ecstatic fever that floated on her skin. The name of Kàrola, the answer it used to have for everything, no longer wanted to respond to your command. Now it's the dead face, the overripe wax mask, panting, stuffed with tubes, that you always see.

But tonight Kàrola spares you oblivion. Yes, it is she who arrives, who infuses your shadow with her glow, the warm woman inside whom all your frost melts. Your flesh is turning like brioche, the afternoon batch baked in the Italian village where she was born and which bears the name of the local pottery. The grain of her skin comes back to you, liquid earth, dancing beneath your lips, the taste of it curling round your molars.

For a long, long time your mouth hasn't watered. But she comes back and the pot of your mouth cracks. Pours forth its waters, weans you from dryness, turns your lips pink. The pain yawns, stretches and goes away. Kàrola is *visiting* you. Grace, recovery, miracle, the words of the catechism come back to you in the height of your hallucinatory dream.

This time you hold the dream, you hold the stressed *kà* of Kàrola, you grasp it and will not let it go.

Yes, it is she who you are following. God, how you love her skeleton – probably the Pò river, bursting its banks, fed her plain? Oh country girl, are you rising from the dead? The flowers around the wells are growing again. Malaria eventually died out.

Yes, it is you, your cheekbones: high, they are very high. They stick out, telling of the slow horde from the East who, crouched behind the smoke of the campfire, suddenly climbed on their animals and went off to overthrow with their cries the immense silence of the 5th century. Country woman from the Pò: Hun, Burgund or Visigoth? What rape of which ancestor, warm woman, has pained you with those cheekbones, slanted your eyes, set wide apart for a calm and confident look?

Woman, my woman, all bronze, all blue. White and pink a little too: your knee or your hipbone – Austrian? – descended from which young girl with golden plaits, terrified of her master's whip, who would have left you some cells from her shaking limbs?

But your hair is blue-black, from the kingdom of the Two-Sicilies. Your armpit is blue like the Southern light, a quiet day in Messina – or Matera? The year 1000 had just begun, the village had ceased to burn. The horses were awaiting their riders (tiny horses with short legs), still trembling from the great sweat.

Kàrola, you held my happiness and I called you 'you'. What infamy from what century of your lineage, what horseless chariots ended their race in your flesh to rot there, as if by accident? You should have been on the watch. Why did you let silence grow until it covered the sound of the alarm? Did I lay my cheek on your belly in vain? Who was the traitor? Are you coming back to make me hear, you who heard nothing?

What do you want of me, my dead one? For I have seen you dead, do you know that now? What do you know of me, calling myself 'you' as though I were someone else? I have seen you dead, my dead one, bloodless, empty, the red soup clotted in your sealed veins. I have seen you dead, my dead one, there, wrapped up in lymph, subtle glue for your broken ligaments. I have seen your satin box, I have seen the oils with which you would anoint it. Show me your nails. Have they grown too long? What dust powders your eyelids? I have dreamed of your urn, you who preferred earth and wood. I have dreamed of covering up your urn. It would be you, a roughly weighed volume of your volatile flesh. It would be you, this regular grain (without even a fragment of charred collarbone). I would dig my fist into it. I would test the residual salt, my breath held behind my cautious lips, my tongue coiled back in terror, I would touch your immanence. And you're stretched out in a box inaccessible to my consciousness, taboo like a spell, like radioactive waste in a canister. So, who *is* this 'you' who 'I' could be ? Who are *you*, Kàrola?

The grace of her visitation fades into a scream.

(The pain that covers your pores makes you realize it's already tomorrow. Sweat, pain and anger have been lying dormant for three hours.)

Marginal Notes: July

I still haven't clarified what drives me to explore her death, and also her after-death and my pre-death. (I acknowledge that this must seem monstrous to you, a dreadful mystification.) But I can't imagine that such an attempt won't also be enlightening and salutary.

If I remember rightly, I have killed all those I have loved, one after the other, over the last 20 years, in some way typical of our times. I enjoyed, while imagining them dead, the sense of terror this anticipated loss brought me. Until the day when, having savoured it enough, I began to hope for it.

This conversion of terrified imaginings into calculated hope always followed the same procedure. I always started by seeing them dead: 'incurable disease' because discovered too late, road or plane accident. I have never imagined electrocution, though I could have. They were unjust deaths, in any case, either because of their brutal suddenness – though people do die suddenly like that, caught in the web of statistics – or through a 'fatal development' that had taken place too early in comparison with contemporary life expectancies.

I can still feel it, this slippage, these dreamy imaginings becoming an imagined wish – held in check by the uncertainty of how it might be fulfilled – that eventually revealed to my consciousness an imminent and irremediable damage: not the physical death of the Other that I thought I wished for, but the emotional death of a love that had ceased to exist and whose human bankruptcy had not yet been declared.

It was in this zone of repression, full of anaesthetized fury, that my sadness grew, through an unspeakable mourning transformed into an imagined mourning. For in fact it was my own death I was imagining in this death of the Other. But at the time I did not know it. (I must have found it too difficult to mourn myself.) Dead to love – or should I simply say to lust? – I thought myself alive enough to be able to kill what was holding me back, and to come to life gain. I eventually understood the process of this murder to be an antidote to the prescribed but always un-predictable, and therefore so much feared, end of our mortal endeavours.

In other words, I preferred to force things. Neither loved nor in love, as long as I could send my dead love to its death, I could watch myself come back to life again. But the relief gained from these deaths was relative. One murder soon leads to another. (That's why the murderers who have died from love, they say, these fathers, these furious lovers, end up killing themselves.) Have I reached this point?

On the one hand, I have started to *see* dying again. Although I thought I was cured of this tendency, I have started once more – in the name of what sense of urgency? – to prefer to force things. On the other hand, it looks as though the death of Kàrola is not enough, that I have to associate with it my own agony rather than my return to life. I hadn't applied the rule of murderers to myself yet. Is this what my cancer inspires me to do?

I say murder and not suicide, which people deplore because it precipitates the hour of death: an illogical complaint since in the end successful suicide coincides with death and conforms strictly to the fate sought by the one who commits suicide. This is very different from murder, which introduces a foreign element to the accomplishment of this fate. Murder really does force things. People who die in car or plane accidents are murdered. People who die of cancer are murdered.

Whereas in an accidental murder, the layers of fog or the breakdown of the reactor are external forces, cancer is an internal force. This is what likens it to suicide, since it seems that one murders oneself.

But I insist: cancer is the murderer, not oneself.

And yet in the writing that projects such a murder, in the description of this dreamed death of 'her' – of which I would be the impossible survivor – I am making the cancer murder me. As the writer, it is I who orders this murder. Am I then, like the cancer, my own murderer?

Why have I chosen cancer again? Probably for the length of time it allows for agony, and therefore for narration, for digging – backwards – through layers of memory. Then, the imaginative charge it bears, its rich, sometimes contradictory, levels that infiltrate so many semiological areas: emotional, clinical, social, hereditary.

It is not a virus, yet cancer is gaining ground like an epidemic, dreaded as a possibility for all of us, like a death – precipitated or rushed – for anyone. It is not contagious, yet it commands the most ordinary and extraordinary of contagions, the fear of dying *of it.*

A vital collapse caused by a terrifying loss, explained in medical terms as the degeneration of cells, I let myself be killed by cancer from her death – that also caused by a cancer, generalised, of course. A common case of a pseudo-contamination – because it cannot be a question of the same cancer – with rich possibilities for investigation. Setting aside the fact that I am inflicting it on myself, this murder is perpetrated in a physical, not an emotional dimension, even if it seems like an empathetic infection. By 'her' death, 'her' physical murder (need I repeat it?), I could only be killed. But why choose to imagine it beforehand? Who is this double whom I call 'you' and whose body I am laying to waste? As the writer, it is a fact, real: I have cancer. (It was announced to me two weeks ago. And it is not something I have chosen.)

OPEN WOUND III

You are sweating. This sweat makes you yell out. You are screaming. You try to recreate the cry of the last dream, but the cube of your room reverberates with a toneless bawling. You stop yelling, in tears. Now you utter the tearful bleats of an undernourished puppy. You can't weep anymore. You stretch your fingers feebly towards the lamp switch. You look at the clock. It's the worst: it's tomorrow but it's still night. Another three hours of night before dawn, for yelling, for sobs you can't even achieve, for being unable to move your bones in the prison of your body.

Now you know the score, you resign yourself to settling into your pain. You inspect your pain, sounding out every atom of its mass. You know how to do that now, how to imagine yourself the ethnologist of this colony that populates your flesh. You know its expansionist customs. You no longer judge its cruelty, you no longer measure its ferocity, no. Calmly you explore the rout of your senses.

Inside, your screams are the continuous bass, almost inaudible, that backs the chorus of your pain. But nothing stands out in this chorus, everything is blended together into the same colourlessness. Grey is often used to mean dull, abandoned. Yet grey is soft, pearly, with velvety blue reflections, a red sheen, grey is such a sweet copulation of blacks and whites. Grey is a true colour in comparison with this non-colour that orchestrates your pain, climbs the bars of your skeleton.

Why, 'my' bones, are you ill?

You have heard the question. Awake, no longer dreaming, you repeat it hesitantly. You listen to the possessive pronoun which has returned to its rightful place. You try to enlarge its territory. I. My bones. I, skeleton. I, tumour. I, dead. My sweat. My death? Why? When?

Slowly you swim upstream to your origin: 'I', born. (You remember the date, indelible from so many Social Security forms.) Awake, no longer dreaming, you try: 'you', 'my' love. Too fast: the live pronouns provoke a groan. 'You', 'my' woman, 'you'. (How to stand firm now 'you' have disappeared?) You try again, pulling yourself up on the broken fragments of your dreams: 'I', attempted in the First Person singular. A load of survival is pulling you from your 'you' of the dead, pushing it to float outside you like an astral body. You try to get up. You are going to try in the First Person. Do 'I' want to? 'I' will try.

But, tied to the shore. (The mooring to the world breaks with this step which fails to support me.) I place my hope in the crystal of the floor, but I fall onto my wobbly knees. I stagger on the distorting glass and sink into its curves. From one room to another, I push through the air, entangled in the harness that keeps me ashore. Hemmed in, I do not call for help. Tottering I set off, condemned, along the pass of the corridor, through the door's portcullis. I tackle the staircase in order to prove it inaccessible. Falling at last, I fall under the force of injust gravity.

Above, the night nurse sleeps peacefully.

Kàrola, I'm going to remember, if you don't mind.

Swimmer, you were swimming. I was watching you. I am watching you. My eyes conjure up the foam, its clear bubbles frothing at the rock of your soft body. My mouth runs smoothly over your dripping shoulder, a mound of cream, the tip of an iceberg. I glimpse your snatching mouth: a cup of air balanced on the pink slide of your windpipe. I stretch open your thorax with a powerful blow, sweet as eternity. Otter, I can swim in the pool of your mucous membranes, swaying with the blows from your heart.

Like a galley, your body, split open by the mad rhythm of the drum, I kiss, neither slave nor mistress, ecstatic from the long-lasting redness.

Oh Kàrola, 'I' no longer know, I no longer know which dream to choose: dying would be a respite. The air is a lead blanket – how to stop that? – the plexus is exhausting my ribs. I used to have healthy bones. But as you see, I can no longer stand firm, alive. You, dead, I can't support no longer supporting you. What about swimming? I would swim, Kàrola, I would board our Cythera, your circled vessel, to the palace of our pink ablutions, of our salty tides. Perhaps.

I remember, my '*dormeuse du val*', I would say *Go!*, blow softly on your darkness so your little folds would dry out to the last bubble. Little stuffed hole, let it breathe a little, let it dry, let it rest. Sea cave, cute cunt, warmth, close in your earthy smell. Last stream, surprise the sheet, last drop, let me sniff you. Your flow has no set course, it is to be lapped up. (I was there.) The forefinger, quickly, pushes the crumb into the hole. Storm of jam.

Instead of that, you are trampling the mists of time. Until what future docking in space?

The window whitens, dawn stretches out in its colourless frame. It is today. The layers of night lose their density, fade away in exhausted slow motion, then come together again, an undifferentiated mass of awakenings and dreams, of consciousness and illusion, as dense as life itself. This *you*, this *she* said over and over, have laid the touchstones for a landscape still unattainable but plausible. A depth of field has been restored by the distance between the 'I' and the exhumed pronouns. No longer plagued with non-existence, but vibrant from their run in the night, returned like an echo in the name of Kàrola, in the stressed *kà* of Kàrola, of *you* Kàrola: 'she'.

Today, I am leaving the house. It was our house.

Marginal Notes: August

I begin to understand what forces me to explore her death – given here as a fact – and my own, trapped in this physical and emotional agony. I no longer need to cover my tracks by imagining that you will consider it monstrous (a dreadful mystification). My conviction that I must exhume what is buried and clarify what is blurred has been strengthened. This is what I call a salutary attempt.

I said – but several days have passed since then – that my cancer was 'announced' to me two weeks ago. I added, 'And it is not something I have chosen.' Today, just as I would no longer deny the emotional nature of the agony represented, I would also no longer write in such a way.

Let's take the first element: I notice that I use the verb 'to announce'.

Cancer, an Annunciation? What myths are we fed on? Does cancer have to be announced, like a birth, a death, a victory? Would it be a victory over both birth and death? And when I was asserting that it was not something I had 'chosen', didn't I mean rather that it was not something I had ever 'hoped for'? No, this hypothesis was still too new.

But today, and it has taken such a short time (cancer has quickly become part of my daily life), I feel inclined to stick to this phrasing: 'Never would I have hoped to have cancer.' Which in everyday language means that I was desperately relying on it, certainly unable to confess as much yet assiduously dreaming of it. This fear of dying *of it* that I mentioned earlier, this fear spreading like a rumour, nurtured by what looks like an epidemic, is experienced in an isolated, fascinated silence. In this silence, temptation is developed, the fear of a major confrontation is prepared and tasted. Hope? (Who has not dreamed of becoming rich?) My hypothesis is that behind the conventional complaints of our mechanical humanity, the magnificent struggle against an announced death has already taken place on a secret inner stage, which prepares us better than we might imagine for the openly dreaded coming. It is like those poverty-stricken lottery winners who become billionaires and who are thought to be uncomfortable with their new wealth, but who adapt overnight to a jet-set lifestyle.

At the risk of ruining myself, but that's another story, here I am *nouveau-riche* from the announcement of my cancer, comfortable as if I fully deserved this 'victory', birth and death together, each enriched by the other, at the heart of my life.

It is breast cancer.

I am formulating it in the narrative present tense, but from the announcement to the confirmation there have been three formulae: this could be cancer, this must be cancer, this is cancer.

(Any cancer, once announced and then confirmed, carries on being described in the present – I have cancer – even when the cancerous tumour has been removed.)

It began with a more or less routine visit to the clinic. In fact, a previous visit had revealed some microcalcifications, recognised as causing a high percentage of malignant developments, which I did not believe for a minute would be the case with me. Out of politeness, but unconcerned, I attended the cancer centre for a 'check-up', my mind absorbed by a conference for which I might be late, my eyes hardly distracted in the waiting room by the other crossing glances: these suggested a process in which I had no part, mine was a waiting which I undertook only by chance and of course only in passing. I frequently consulted my watch as though I already had one foot outside the door, certainly not belonging in the anxious interior of a cancer centre.

The doctor, a beautiful woman, tired, did not explicitly affirm what her hand had confirmed. She probably thought I was in too much of a hurry, too much absorbed to absorb the announcement in real time. My irritation at the idea of having to stop work, necessary for the removal of this thing which 'could be' suspect (Do you want to operate?) made her realise that I would only understand alone, once alone, what lay behind her words. Four days later, when I came back to have the pre-operative tests, I had understood.

From then on, I was, I was to be, part of this process in the waiting rooms that I had scarcely glanced at a few days earlier.

Cancer could be announced.

The confirmation of the malignancy, after the lumpectomy, through a biopsy (I have become familiar with the jargon) was no more than a formality.

But I would like to examine to this notion of familiarity, not only with the medical jargon I was absorbing with disconcerting ease, despite my lack of scientific training, but with cancer, which as I said above quickly became part of my daily life. Could I compare this feeling with that of an athlete who, after a remarkable performance which gained him a medal that turned him into a demi-god, claimed not to be 'surprised' by his new status, was not absolutely amazed, once the trauma of victory had worn off?

If I pursue this metaphor, might I compare my life to a long preparation, an intensive training – punctuated by failures and disappointments – until this victory, like walking through a mirror, brings me into the familiar, satisfied, peaceful world of a fulfilled dream?

Then what do I do with the slow, virulent process of murder which confronts me on walking through the mirror? Have I already forgotten the cost of this passage? What is this becalmed sea where I find myself taking down the mast as if the worst (an ordinary, unchosen fight) was behind me?

Here I am, chosen. I am told that the fight, the real fight, lies ahead, but I am looking up at the sky, floating, lying in the bottom of my boat. ('The harmonious ether, with its azure waves, wraps the mountains in a purer fluid.') Out of this minimalist azure, released from minor worries, suddenly appears the real stage where I am going to act out, where I am already acting out, with some obscure talent, my horror of death.

Though I display a remarkable energy and remain vigorous – I am a very healthy woman – in the aftermath of the operation and its train of treatments, though I show a docile optimism in the course of everyday exchanges, my clandestine writing is an inventory of the agony of my bones, of my life. I have always known that bone cancer could develop from breast tumours. (A piece of fiction always has its own logic.)

OPEN WOUND IV

Fearful shaking. On the motorway the ambulance they sent skidded on the wet road. I was frightened. (I am tracing the trickles of foam.) I was frightened and I am frightened. Listen to my heartbeat, it's hiccoughing. (How to stop such a rain?) The hospital is still 10 minutes away.

This morning I put on my stockings and my summer shirt, renounced the night. They closed the shutters of the house. I was very cold – my soul in tears, and so heavy on the stretcher.

I said, Don't close all the shutters, leave those in the bedroom.

My plexus restrains the hiccoughing of my heart. I trace the foam, the flurries on the liquorice strip of the road. And now 'I' want to live. I could feel this morning that I didn't want to still, that I already wanted to. I said, Yes, treat me, take me, don't close all the shutters, it was our house.

Listen: at the break of dawn I opened the drawer and pulled out my notebook. There I breathed in the smell of after my death. (It smelled of the small writing desk in my mother's bedroom.) It wasn't just the smell it gave off, it was the permanence, already, of an unchanging mould settled in the spine of this prematurely yellowed book. I put the book down, raised it again to my nostrils. I lapped the thread that bound the opened pages, was reminded of my peeling skin, breathed it in deeply. The salt, so close, this regular grain (without even a fragment of charred collarbone).

That was before my death. Oh, how I would like to smell no stronger than these succulent leaves, this dry aroma etched on the cover. At last I would be at peace, wrapped in the pages, stuck with my own glue. Later, the spine would dry out. Much later, the stickiness of the stains.

See: I had become used to sweat, to pain. I had become used to my murder, to agony. I thought that agony was like death, I wished it so.

I was waiting. I had to die. I had become used to it. I waited. And then, you see, this fearful shaking, my familiar fear of the rain, of a car accident. It is a naïve fear. Now my blood is starting to run quickly again like when I was young and survived an attempt at water-skiing. (It was the first time I came within an ace of death.) But does one die at 20?

Tell me: what is this love that has ruined my bones? I can no longer live with it, but, living, I would like to stay so, I would like to grow a little older, to hop up with each chirp of the grasshopper. What unexpected doubt is encircling the too-late, for it is too late, isn't it? You are saying: you should have said so earlier. Did it have to be said?

Echoes of my last night, as dense as life, the sound of the wind creeping around the house, climbing like a vine, a hungry dream where I called her 'you', chill awakening where I named her 'she', and this screaming fury where I tried the 'I', the 'you', as if it had to be kept alive by being said over again.

They came to collect me, my soul in tears, and so heavy on the stretcher. I repeated, It was our house, don't close all the shutters, leave those in the bedroom.

I wanted to live then.

But here is the hospital. Saved?

Marginal Notes: September

I had seen myself on the brink of grasping what I am pursuing by writing about my death and hers – I might as well call her Kàrola, her name could nearly be Kàrola – but all of a sudden I feel threatened by the narration, overwhelmed by a progression in which my double takes over, somehow preempted by her own salutary attempt. As for me, I can't see anything enlightening in it, and the 'harmonious ether' I was examining from the bottom of my boat stinks of the stench of the hospital. Far from ordering anything at all, I have become the servile handmaid of my real cancer. Now writing about it seems monstrous, and the style a dreadful mystification.

Let's sum up. My name is Jacqueline J. (I refuse to give my double my own name.) I won't let her borrow my life, my sweat, my pain. I refuse my involvement with the existence of this one who is dying, this 'cancer of the bones', this irresolute 'metastasis' that might be real or imagined, we don't know. If Kàrola's – her metastasis – is dead, she is the one who has dreamed it, not I. Or someone else is writing through us. (Can I believe this?)

So I should fear my cancer – of course, dying *of it*, everyone is expecting it, aren't they? – but it is Kàrola's death – mine, the real one – that terrifies me. Knowing that she is exposed to the risk of losing me, I feel exposed to her loss, to the misinterpretation of my past and present evil spells, turned round like the dangerous curses of an apprentice witch.

Not only is my cancer trying to murder me, but it is rummaging through the rubble of a room expressly closed. Like a vulture, my conscience offers it the candle. Silence, I say, I want silence, I want the shadow of silence.

My hair has started to fall into my hand. It is falling, sad tufts escaped from my crown. I look at my dethroned eyes. Nothing can be read in my eyes. That's the problem: where is the sign that I've walked through the mirror? I thought I was satisfied, lying in the bottom of my boat. The real fight lies ahead – or so they tell me – but I can't see any fight where I must clash swords. My 'salutary' fervour, my 'enlightening' attempts, all that was probably just the provision of fresh cells from which I benefited for a while. Today, and already for some time, I have got into the habit of – I almost said I'm inhabited by – no longer being alone.

All this fiction, do you think I'm in charge of it? The framework has escaped my control and I have no desire to retrieve it. Let the one who is dying slip away if that's what she wants, let her come back to life again – such miraculous remissions have been known, they do occur – let her forget her love, dead or alive, let her fight, if she understands that verb.

My veins are sucking. This is my fight, laid on the stretcher. I suck in liquids that are deadly to my deadly cells. (But did you know that cancer cells are by nature immortal?) So if the fight that is taking place is to the death, it occurs outside of me, without my participation.

I told you, I am no longer alone, and pretending to address an audience is one of the symptoms of my dispossession. By the way, I have noted that my double was beginning to get a taste for it too. I presume that the vocative brings her back into the world. I am not interested.

This is an extremely aggressive carcinoma T2N0 – QSE of the right breast. Its histology is Grade III. A complementary mastectomy is recommended justified by the high risk of local recurrence, after 6 successive chemotherapy treatments (Protocol FEC 50).

When I eat, nothing is as it should be. It isn't a mouth that chews and swallows anymore, it isn't an oesophagus that conveys the mouthful, it isn't a stomach that stirs the juices over a low heat, no, these are other organs, Martian organs, adapted to refuse such little tasks, which change their mind, turn everything upside down and throw up one or more programming errors.

The hospital waiting rooms are now places that form part of my life. I show a real competence there, you can see it in my eyes when they cross less practised glances. They don't know what is in store for them.

I do know. Of course, I can recognise others who are competent: in other glances, this way of being inhabited, in the habit. A sense of being at ease with the secret, a politeness in the anger.

And, everywhere, a tremendous docility.

Never. Never did I think I would become docile. Here is what I expected. At the outset, the removal of a tumour in the right breast (diameter: 4 cm) whose malignancy was confirmed (I have already mentioned the Annunciation). As soon as it was 'removed', I would no longer have cancer. I would have had cancer. I had had cancer.

For safety's sake the area would be swept clean with X-rays, over the time span of a summer. Later, much later, I would have to say, being careful about the tense, concentrating on thwarting any attempt at pity, I have had cancer in my right breast.

Instead of this, which would have been a swift clash of swords, a daring tilt at a jauntily held banner – considering the process, the ceremony of the waiting rooms, the liturgy of outpatients whose rituals I have absorbed so well – instead of this rapid fight, I have seen myself pushed to the heart of a severe and persistent conflict. And, above all, deadly boredom.

I envied my double her agony. In the very abandonment of her life, I could see the construction, the mastering and the completion of a project. I envied the autonomy of her project. But then, resistant, overseer of a territory mined by myself, she is capable of launching – to my own confusion – a mine-clearing operation.

In the conflict into which the generals in white have thrown me – they promised I would be on the front line – I am bored, I have submitted to the docility demanded by their protocol. I am bored by this conflict. The generals have taken over the official strategy and stake of the battle – the safeguarding of my mined territory – but that is their only concern. What do they care about my soil, its beauty, its fertility, what do they care about the grain of the crust of my earth, the fire it is holding? All they are concerned about are the terrorists, as they call them, who inhabit my domain. My soil is their battleground and therefore is no longer the ground of my resistance.

Docile, I let them pound my domain.

I envied my double her project of agony. In what is happening to her, as in a *volte face*, I find myself as helpless as in the face of a betrayal in which I do not want to believe, but which destroys my certainty. In the contrary project in which she is engaged, without my knowledge and almost by accident, I sense a dangerous plan, a new monstrosity with extraordinary consequences. Nothing prepared me for this.

Did I have to be fully alive, to write, to dream of death! Today, bored to death, all plans of victory given over to my generals, I restrict my competence to the practice of submission. I put down any burst of rebellion and even consent to the betrayal of my double. Long may she live if that's what she wants. But no loud excitement, no cries of jubilation, let everything slip quietly by, as it already has, without my knowledge. And let them give me some sleeping tablets.

OPEN WOUND V

The Regional Centre for the Fight against Cancer provides patients with 630 staff chosen for: their special training; their particular qualifications; their human qualities. The medical team gathers in a single location 110 doctors, all specialists in one or more of the different related disciplines. The permanent pooling of their competencies ensures the best possible management of the disease ...

The R.C.F.C. is entitled to receive donations and legacies, tax-deductible for the donators ... A technical panel noted for its achievements ... enables the implementation, without delay, of treatments whose early administration improves their efficacy.

Good morning Madame how are we doing this morning? That colour really suits you (Don't worry I'm just giving you an injection in preparation for the scan.) I love mauve too (Someone will come and get you in half an hour.) My mother says it reminds her of mourning – what an idea I say no one dresses in mourning anymore mauve is elegant it suits brunettes as well as blondes don't you think? (Let me know if I'm going too fast.) Mauve, you're blonde and that suits you *really* well (...) Look, your hair is growing back. (That's it you're ready someone will come and get you in half an hour.)

Medical Liaison Notebook

You are presently at the R.C.F.C. and are being treated with a chemotherapy adapted to your disease. This treatment might cause side-effects, such as disorders caused by the toxicity of the medication to the bone marrow. The respective attack of the white corpuscles, platelets, red corpuscles can be a source of infections, bleedings, anaemia ... During your treatment at the Centre, if there are some foods that disagree with you, please do not hesitate to ask for a dietician to help you to adapt your meals to your tastes.

Dream Notebook

Usual ripples at starting the first page. A wave of little 'me's, ready to leap, inflate my abdomen. Writing, writing the truth, nothing is more difficult. An application at the most: the wave grows bigger, and smaller. Crashes on the foamy ground which it left behind when it retreated.

Nothing granite-like.

What a modest task it is to write only in the present when one would like *the end*. To know, wanting to know how it will end, but having nothing but this gift of crumbs. The wave of little 'me's inflates, grows bigger, grows smaller, would like. Willing. Unwilling. Nothing serious.

I should write down the dates, I would just have to ask the nurses, What day is it today? And then I would be able to count one day after the next. I would ask again when I was no longer sure. There wouldn't be anything extraordinary about that, losing count, in a captive daily life. But is that what I'm looking for, is the order of the days necessary, in this speaking the underside? For whom?

To claim each day to transcribe the other side of my speaking the outside is certainly an illusion. Not wanting to say anything more about appearances, it is as though I was deciding to descend to the soft fire of the Earth without travelling through the crust. Nothing to hang on to. No landscape, no familiar lie. Only this molten rock, below, unbearable to exist in, that I deny as I seek it out, swiftly running away from me. The underside. What is the underside? And the underside of what?

Violence. To write the truth is nothing but violence.

N. and A. have given me this notebook, convinced that I will be able to write something important now that I'm getting better. But from one sentence to the next, from one paragraph to the next, I retain nothing. I'm reluctant to reread to see if there's anything I might learn from it, suspicious of my propensity for evasion, sure or nearly sure of finding nothing but empty babble.

I walked today. And it wasn't a dream.

What has just been written here? A speaking of the surface. The language of a ship's log. As if I had completely forgotten my feeble decision: to write, only, the underside of my voice, of appearances, to write, not a soliloquy to the winds, but the cautious probing of my lie. What did I think I would discover? What did I expect to live through when dying?

All the same, I really should make a note of this: today (the same ones) have brought me a dictaphone, a toy, a small, black, smooth receiver I can hold in my hand. Their intention was for me to rediscover the desire, the distance desire imposes, to start speaking. I was very frightened. To travel, alone, through the knotted crust of my voice! As if everything had to be said! I've put the black toy in the bottom of the drawer. Speaking exhausts me. But to write, to dream, isn't that exhausting too?

My dreams, every night, continue their voyage to unattained destinations. Without ever managing to retain the points of the journey, I nevertheless remain impregnated with the incompleteness of the quest outlined within.

Never soothed, always diverted.

I am looking after some very beautiful cats that run away. I look for them, anguished, randomly. I find others, awfully appealing. I would so much like it to be them that I was responsible for and that I've allowed to escape. I would like to be able to swap them, though I know full well that they are not interchangeable. The dream ends without a solution. It's a nightmare. I wake up to the swift oblivion of relief from my wanderings, gnawed at by a thousand contingencies. I remain struck, though, by a similarity between the dream and the awakening. I know they have something in common, but what?

How to descend to the soft fire without travelling through appearances, the sumptuous crust of the green valleys? And why green, why want valleys to be green? What about their faults, their mass of fallen earth? Kàrola, yes, Kàrola was a green valley. That is what I used to see. But haven't I seen it all?

Marginal Notes: October

I haven't much to add. My double is having a good time. She writes and speaks on my behalf, although she claims it exhausts her. She manages the terrors that still assault her well, and I have no doubt that she triumphs over the rocks in the current where I drop my anchor. Mauve suits her and her hair is growing back. The last bone scan she had confirmed a halt in the proliferation of her 'playful' cells.

I bow before the monstrous depths into which she has been dragged and I hope that her predicted rise – salutary, of course – brings her the enlightenment she desires. Unless this is another mystification? For my part, I would regard that as dreadful, and I assert that I no longer want anything to do with this existential bawling.

Of course, the evidence is against me. I claimed myself to be orchestrating this agony – this murder? – confused but certain to find a meaning in it, a truth. Did I feel as I have claimed as strong, as clever as my cancer? It was a mistake. Cancer has the cleverness all murderers have, and while my unharmed cells are growing older, while my brain cells are dying – short life – its immortal cells have their own eternity.

Its attempted murder of my double was not the result of an order from me (how could I believe that?) but the effect of its labour of death within me. So I would like to understand, in this dubious set-up, why the remission of this Other, whom I call my double, rather than comforting me, weighs me down. Seeing her occupied once more in seeking out the truth, I feel furious that I can't find it anywhere, I'm envious of her pathetic attempts. Here she is, seeking out, yes, beneath the crust, the fault where the lie might have crept in. She is an agony ahead of me. Strong in the hope of living again, she has every opportunity to question what was lying in her dying. I, crippled with the fear of dying, have no interest in seeking out what is lying or was lying in my living. Perhaps the emotional paralysis to which my generals have brought me makes me intolerant. But how to get them to understand that their superficial war, their strategy of scorched earth, gives me no access to the soft fire, to the faults masked by the beautiful crust. Here she is, the Other, ready to question the luxuriance of her desire. As for me, the confession is out of my reach. And I feel furious that she, so close to me, is so close to it.

Can we, she and I, meet in the same epicentre? I see her, leaning over the tip of the crater, ready, close to spotting the fault, ready, close to doubting the visible beauty.

For a long time I have been resting in this landscape of beauty and fault. Of course, the peace I found there is still there, though threatened. I have already described it, in old notebooks where I thought I was looking for purity, the 'green valley' as school-children call it, for snow 'the white coat'.

I knew it so well, the tawdriness of the well-turned phrase, the nice, sweet epithets that speak of something else: green valley to say happiness, peace, quiet cat or dog in the sun, absence of or forgetting the war, the last one or the one to come. Only the ordinary rape of mothers by their husbands coming back from the fields. Green valley for patri-rural civilisations, at the expense of a stabbing per minute.

Today, to write about the crust or the fire it is holding, to write is nothing but violence. I force into it the shards of a deficient pronunciation, that of my tongue slowed down by a brain reluctant to show its underside.

Oh purity, what impurities there are beneath your bell jar!

I don't know how to get out of this. I had this desire to describe a perfect arch. The transfer of the open wound to the very flesh of another self, the murder of her very bones. The extrapolated death, projected outside the frame of my terror. (What clearing up I hoped for, on the cheap.)

But I can see myself confused as much by the unforeseeable – but unavoidable – twist in my narration, as by the twist in these notes.

Is this the work of someone with cancer?

Let's sum up. Didn't I say that as a writer I liked to take cancer as a model? I thought this was right: isn't cancer the most elaborate attempt at substituting one reality for another? (As such, it appears the archetype of creation.) But my ignorance was equalled only by my boastfulness. These cancerous cells are playing by the rules of another game and care nothing for the Creation. Like a lie – that spreads through our relationships, our ambitions, our silences – cancer weaves the most extraordinary simulacrum. Meanwhile the cells of our conscience are dying – a short life. In fact, they are dying of fear, cowardice, loneliness. Killing the cancer doesn't kill the lie.

This is what the generals cannot understand. They fight against a symptom, believing that they are curing the disease. They kill the terrorists in the bush. The bush is burning. But where have the terrorists come from? Does the cure mean that we will never know? Where will we find the tracks of truth on the scorched earth?

Today cancer is as much a part of me as my skin, as my organs poisoned by the venom used to try to wipe it out. Today cancer takes the place of truth for me. This murderer and companion has dispatched its playful cells to that place, has annexed the territory of the unconfessable. From that moment on, my cure could only be a new metaphor for a lie. It would be at odds with the meaning and origin of such an annexation.

For cancer knows well the land it has conquered. This is why it is so familiar to me and takes the place of truth for me. Within this context I understand why my double's self-redemptive manoeuvres irritate me so much. Who does she think she's fooling? Cancer came. Driven out, if a 'cure' of some sort can possibly drive it out, it will take our secrets with it. It is up to us whether we want to live with this knowledge: that cancer is dead and the lie alive. The growing awareness of this dissimulation does not seem to bother my double. Of course, she's thinking: 'Haven't I seen it all?' Earlier, cursing, this is how she addressed her dead one: 'Have you come to make me hear, you who heard nothing?'

Come on, neither she nor I saw or recognised the lie, the soft fire that was smouldering beneath the crust. We were not able to see or recognise the tumour of the lie. Our generals, intent on wiping out the tumour, believe that they are killing the disease, but as I said before: they are deluding themselves with a symptom, called cancer.

OPEN WOUND VI

Dream Notebook

I am taking up this notebook again after a long interruption. (I don't have time to explain why.) This morning, in the mirror, *I looked at myself*, for a long time, aware of the conventions of this face to face, but determined to persist. In fact, the two of us were summoned. In answering this summons, something had to happen between us, standing there, in front of and behind the mirror. We touched my hair, real hair. We ran our hands over my face, which I had just made up. Our eyes questioned this make-up of the living, both standing there, in front of and behind the mirror. A residual thinness about the cheekbones emphasised the lines of our outlined eyelids. The mouth, motionless, was silent. A harmony began to show itself on our withered skin. A silence.

It is this silence I come from, it might be this silence that has summoned us, silence, at last, between her and me. (Between the lie and me? Between death and me?)

I had delegated to death its task, and here I am alive only to live. It is very little, in fact, there is very little to do. But having taken on death's share of the task, I still feel excessively tired, as after an over-long journey. (It is not a matter for regret, we all make mistakes.)

I can no longer get my thoughts going again, as if they have been slowed down by my possible cure. The cure saturates my words. The disease was talkative, loquacious, delved into everything. My desire was dead, but death *was* my desire. There was a lot to do. Cured, I have to relearn the round of small, everyday mortal wants. Cancerous and anguished, I sought immortality. It was an immoderate ambition. It was a dreadful mystification. But it was, also, the truth.

She who is writing invented Kàrola's murder and, like cancer – her cancer – has tried to murder me. How right she was (a piece of fiction always has its own logic): I could only be killed by the murder of my desire. I understand her fear of renewing her old murderer's tendencies, but those were nothing more than early drafts born out of sincerity. Her new attempt, which she so much hoped would be 'enlightening' and 'salutary', was in fact an attempt at this 'unconfessable confession': the death of desire, turned into the desire for death, into a cancerous tumour. Cancerous, I have embodied desire, death. Dying, I have embodied the unconfessable mourning of desire.

When will she accept the truth she has created herself, out of our crazy cells? When will she realise that we are each the same and the Other for the author of this text?

Alive, cured perhaps, back soon to the little burdens of everyday life, she, I, whom she calls her double, are returning to our homonymous ways. A little crushed by her fiction, which was the truth only so long as it was unveiled, we will now have to play the game, to end victorious in the war led by those she calls her generals, be cured, with docility, by their victory, which is *their* victory. Does the Other who writes really know what she's doing by writing about us like this? Didn't the lethal disease in her desire raise other questions that she will have to answer with other doubles? Who is going to be cured in the end? Who is responsible for the cure?

For it is about responsibility, being about a cure. So heavy with her memory of death. So tired. So tired of questioning. Who betrayed whom? Who murdered what?

Let's sum up. The Other thought it a good idea to write the fiction of her probable death, born of Kàrola's death, given as a fact. She didn't know how well she did. Here she is, caught in the trap of her own attempt. I am now a dreamed agony ahead of her in expressing the confession she thinks herself incapable of making, cornered by the lie of her pretence. Is she going to carry on pretending for long?

Cured, that is to say, lucid about the lie of a cure when the truth of the disease is masked, now I would like to describe only landscapes, valleys. I will be the inhabitant of these valleys, green valleys. Inhabited by me, by Kàrola. I would be looking after cats which I wouldn't lose. My numerous friends would present me with numerous gifts on my return. They would celebrate my new state of body, which would correspond to my state in fact: Amazon. I would be the Amazon who aims at her desire. Come on, what would be this target of my desire? What belongs to us, once we are cured?

Marginal Notes: November

What I finally realise, in the exhaustion of my tongue in these marginal notes, is that here the cure of my cancer is being played out, here it lies. I thought I had transferred the worst on to my narration. I tried to suck the cancer from the inside, strictly applying its murderer's method. I made all its lethal, stupid cells proliferate (condensation of as many confessed deliriums as unconfessable confessions …). I set my double all the traps, I poured into her my despair at having lied, at not having been able to create sincerity except in the making of my tumour.

I understand better now why cancer became the only 'truth' at my disposal. I understand better now the meaning of my October revolt. At least the disgust I felt for my servility gave me back my taste for freedom.

Leaning over the lip of the crater, I can see myself ready, close to spotting the fault, ready, close to recognising my unique terror, my fundamental terror: not that I may be mortal, but that I may be dead to desire.

I wished so much that desire might be immortal. I wished so much for the immortality of its cells. 'An end to everything, except desire.' This diktat in stone, sprayed amusingly on the

walls of Paris, haunts me. And I am exhausted by this bitter suspicion: which of the two of us will live the longest? As always, it is a
question of the only thing capable of binding or unbinding lovers:
the truth, the said truth, the truth said. To be said . . . now? Right
away? Not necessarily. But not much later, just before 'too late'.
What a stake, what a training for a tightrope-walker. What fear of
dragging down the other in a vertigo, in a fall. What currents
ready to sweep me along are still hidden beneath this fear?

Are you scared, yes or no, asks the lover? The answer today is
no. But I 'made' a cancer. Does that mean I was scared yesterday?
Does that mean I was unloving? What merit, unknown to me,
will triumph in the end? Perhaps this narration, who knows. I
wrote, though the meaning of what I was writing escaped me. I
couldn't know what 'I' wanted to say. Perhaps I believed for a
while – that was in July, I still had an abundance of healthy cells –
that my jabbering in the margin would capture what I couldn't
work out (and what was frightening me) in this vertigo of an
agony set in the present tense.

In these soliloquies in the margin, thank God in the margin, I at
last flush out my blatant offences of amnesia: but going back over
the gaps in the work of the past is in no way an antidote to the
anaerobic 'viruses' that are still smouldering, ready to emerge
should the opportunity arise. That's it. I know it now. It's an
emotional and physical knowledge. My fictional double – dear
double – taught me more about lying than my so-called quest for
truth. Soon, I hope, we will meet again in the same epicentre. But
first, this breast has to be removed. A mere formality?

OPEN WOUND VII

(*Transcription of my voice*)
The house, I have come back to the house. I've had all the shutters
opened, except those in the bedroom that were open already. I looked at
the bed of my sweat, of my pain. I saw Kàrola waiting for me in the

garden. She had hung out the washing. What a beautiful dead one, my 'dead one', now the lie is dead. (I am dreaming, I am getting everything confused, like the living do.) I choose what I look at, what I listen to. I am cured. I can drink milk, wine, I can smoke long menthol cigarettes, I can sleep on my side beside Kàrola. Not yet face down, not quite. I smell the soft, dry pillow, clear of hair. My hair stays on my head. It is unaware of its youth. It doesn't know yet which way to grow, it knows nothing about me, it is different hair that I don't know. I have abandoned my face to the mirror. It is a good image. I'm certainly a few years older. I don't know how old. No, really, I don't know. I'm all ages, having experienced the age of dying. The generals are pleased with themselves. They say they are pleased with me. They have removed a breast, not the liver. And this suits me, Amazon. And my bones keep my body standing firm, or sitting, which is wonderful. I walk in the valley. Kàrola walks in front of me or behind me, depending. She matches my pace, she doesn't interfere with my tipsy steps. I see her standing aside to let me pass when the path is narrow. I do what the living do: I walk and I come back when the chill air hits my neck. (It just takes a shiver to make you feel alive!)

Tomorrow some friends will come and collect me and we will drive to a painted grotto, recently discovered nearby. We will go and see the traces of the eyes that guided ancient hands, ancient women who lived here, at a time impossible to imagine. On our way back we will stop at a café in a small town where the hot chocolate is as good as in our lost childhood. We will look at the men and women around us. There will be some children too, probably a dog and perhaps a diffident cat. You should see how alive they are, these men, these women, these children who talk and laugh at every little thing as if they possessed immortality all to themselves. Death strikes differently in small villages. Didn't you know that? I know it. It's my grandmother, I think, who told me.

My grandmother, when she went out, always wore a fine shawl and a purple veil. To blow her nose, she would pull out of her black handbag a large striped mauve handkerchief that smelt of lavender water. It's a smell that made me a little sick, but it was my grandmother, one of her smells. Until they put her in her coffin, she smelt of lavender soap. The satin paddings were mauve, coherent. As a young girl I saw death like that, mauve and lavender.

(*Interruption*: The cat, returning from its inspection of the hen house, asked me what I was doing and if I wanted to go out again with it to bring in the washing.)

I don't know what I was saying, about mauve (which suits me so well), my grandmother's lavender water that made her death smell so good. I am going to stop here anyway, it was a first attempt for my unknotted voice in the smooth black receiver. A new game where I am going to learn to speak again, that is to say, to speak better than before, desire, without spoiling things.

Tonight I will put a date in my dream notebook, just to end it, before perhaps beginning another. What to say at the end? Fiction and reality overlap and complement one another. There is no fiction without reality, it is part of it. In writing, we are creating reality through fictions that come out of reality. The afternoon is about to end. The wind is rising. Tonight it will surround the house, creeping like an animal wanting to get in. I can hear the neighbour nailing something together. I have had cancer.

EPICENTRE: DECEMBER

My beloved,

I have just finished this strange piece 'Sweat', started, as you know, well before they 'announced' my cancer. First I want to tell you that I am sorry for having imagined your adored body dying, sorry for having extracted the fiction of your death from the reality of my being alive, sorry, finally, to have fed this dreamed fiction with my own collapse. Initially I didn't know that such a thing would be written. Perhaps the death I thought I could get close to, untouched, and confront with my anticipated horror, with my deferred anger, was already at work in my 'playful' cells.

I would believe anything! I dreamed of exorcising everything, in those paragraphs about my agony, while I was inspired – but why *at this very moment*, years later? – by the terrible agony of Denise. (Denise whom you never knew, but I told you, didn't I, that I loved her like a sister?) And so, 'at this very moment', years later, unaware that I was cancerous myself, I transposed her rotting body into our beloved flesh.

With each invented word – with what atrocious jubilation – I was asking your forgiveness, and I was asking myself why, but the reason escaped me and I went on with this vertiginous mix of illusion and reality (Denise was rotting alive, can you understand?), of desire and repression, writing for myself and against myself, looking for the meaning and the meaning escaping. Then the cancer *came*. My consciousness didn't hope for it that much. But consciousness is always fed by the unconscious, like a skin renewing itself from the inside. My consciousness, finally, was about to be well fed, and the said truth, the truth said, could at last be expressed. It wasn't without its problems. The invasion of truth was so strong that I had to resort to a split personality to give myself some relief.

It is the only trick I could find to express without exhausting myself the exhausting dialectic between the desire to die and the fear of dying *of it*, between self-love and self-hatred, between disease and cure.

As you can see, I am not grouping each term of this dialectic with its respective opposite, a supposed 'positive' or 'negative'. The exhaustion comes from this: the progression of the cure does not necessarily correspond with a sincere expression of self-love. (Sometimes the disease is much more sincere.) And self-love does not dry up the desire for death.

As for desire for the lover, this delightful invasion, how many fantasies of murder does it fail to repulse in the fear that it might be mortal and betray us? I experienced so many mortal desires before you came. And I have betrayed so often and I have so often been betrayed. And I have wept so long at the mortality of my dead desires. And I have fed my mortal desires so long with fantasies of murder. I thought it would be better to end it like that, I thought I would come back to life better, if I murdered my desires before they died. (Even non-cancerous, I was almost aware of this.)

And then I 'made' a cancer, breast cancer. It is such a sincere disease. My breast fed so much of my desire before you with its lies.

My generals have removed my breast, but it is not by removing this breast that they have cured me, and it is not by removing my tumour that they have cured this cancer of accumulated lies. If I am cured, it is from knowing that my desire for you, my beloved, is no more immortal than I am. No more than you are. I am talking about a physical knowledge, discovered with hindsight, buried in the 'sincerity' that the playful cells of my lie have created, through an organic mediation, no doubt elaborated unbelievably.

Which of the two of us will live the longest? No, I will not answer with 'What does it matter?', a phrase whose false elegance betrays once more the lie that always tempts the most sincere love. Sometimes I want you to die first, to 'know' if I could survive it – and it is this vertigo, as a writer, that I have enjoyed exploring, assured that the depths I would lean over into would show me the faults in the beautiful crust. Sometimes I would prefer to die first myself, revealing my narcissistic need to have you close to me 'for ever' (where my pathetic need for infinity can be seen again).

It is then that I wonder about the mortality of your desire, you, my young woman: there is no doubt that you could survive my death. No doubt that you would be able to discover another desire than the one that fills you today.

I am cured not of doubt – the bitter suspicion – but of the invasive terror of doubt. This is what I am cured of, my beloved. And I ask you to forgive me my past lies, my possible future lies, and my present sincerity.

You are not the one through whom the cancer came, you are the one with whom the cancer was cured. Oh, I have been scared, do you know that?, not of dying *of it*, but of losing my desire. It was so exhausting, this position, leaning over the edge of the fault.

Today, in front of you, I appear whole, asymmetrical, in the beauty of my restored truth which I present to you. With this gift, I am ending the notebooks of my sweat, of my pain, topsy-turvy recital of my childish dream, the secret passenger I have always carried with me: the desire to love and be loved, for ever.

So, my beloved, you will know that I have chosen you again, not for a forever charged with death, but for a today laden with the most precious load: our life.

To you, my beauty, I dedicate my new Amazon's body, capable of knowledge.

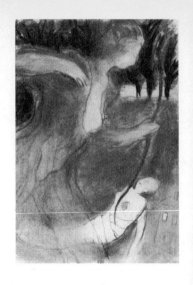

Diana

For Catherine Arthur

CATHERINE RAE ARTHUR: ANOTHER WAY OF SEEING

Dale Gunthorp

Catherine Arthur didn't intend her cancer drawings to be seen as 'art'. They were, she insisted, only an attempt to work something out. In fact, during their making, she didn't want them to be seen at all. Catherine was always wary of the loud voice of the outside world, which made it difficult for her to hear her own. This quest for quiet, for contact with a reality just out of view, ran through all her life. She dreamed of living in a room with one window, one table, plate and fork, one blanket and one picture on the wall. She loved the bare line, the fugitive colour. She saw elements of herself in such artists as Gwen John, Mark Rothko and the poet Emily Dickinson. She returned, again and again, to the anonymous medieval poem, 'The Wanderer', the story of a knight whose lord is dead, who roams through a stormy winter landscape, about to perceive the happiness which had before been invisible to him, through his exile from it.

Yet the self that Catherine was made the stillness she sought difficult to achieve. Catherine was spectacularly beautiful. She was witty and socially accomplished. She was clever. Her essays, poems and drawings were pounced on with delight. She could not escape notice. When she had it, she enjoyed it. But she found it false.

Catherine was born in Toronto in April 1937, the eldest of four children in a close, isolated and cold upper-middle-class Anglican family. Through her childhood, she had phases of angelic behaviour interspersed with periods of wild and near-delinquent reaction. She was, however, consistent in being the one member of the family able to stand up to her father's rages and, until she left home at 16, she was the protector of her mother and siblings. Later, she put herself through an honours degree in French literature at the University of Toronto.

In 1963, she left Canada, making her way to England on a Norwegian fishing boat. She came, she said, in search of the world of Jane Austen. She found cold, squalid London, a job as a photojournalist with the Tourist Board and the Sloane gay scene. In parallel with her tumultuous social life, she pursued her quest for that other just-out-of-view reality. She took instruction to enter the Catholic Church, wrote poetry, and filled dozens of A4-sized sketch pads with drawings.

Her career, too, advanced. She was always interested in printing: particularly typography, but also in the whole process from paper-making to bookbinding, and in techniques from calligraphy and hand-setting to the most sophisticated of printing technologies. She moved into technical journalism, becoming editor of *British Printer*, and then features editor of *Printing World*, the leading magazine in this field. During her illness, she took on the editing of *The Quickprinter*, the journal of the association of print and copyshops, and transformed it from a trade news sheet into a stylish and information-packed glossy.

All the while Catherine was also developing her art. She visited dozens of exhibitions every year, attended life-drawing classes, and worked at her drawing. She felt, however, that she would never be able to realise her full potential while she remained a largely untutored weekend painter. In 1985, she took the plunge and reversed the order of her work: she gave up her career for a precarious life of freelance journalism, and began a full-time course at art school. Her work had long been admired for its imaginative richness and elegance of line. At Hornsey, she developed a vigorous, harder style, and learned to work in oils, at a large scale, and to use colour. She found that her views on art were profoundly different from those prevailing in the college: she did not think of painting as self-assertion, political statement or sexual *double entendre*, but as discovery – contact with that other reality. So while she benefited from the technical training, she found the experience aesthetically numbing. She remained interested in what her fellow students and tutors were doing, but followed her own path, undertaking a series of oils and etchings with disturbing images of her 50-year-old self trying to squeeze back into the world of her childhood or, with childlike, wide-eyed curiosity, observing the decay of the body.

Less than a year after her graduation, Catherine discovered a lump in her breast; within a week this had been diagnosed as a malignant cancer, and week by week after that there were further revelations: spread through the lymph nodes, into the spine, and then to other bones. After a year, it began to colonize the soft tissues, the bodily organs. Cancer – the cold disease – is always frightening, but it can be relatively gentle in its depredations. Catherine faced a prognosis of physical breakdown, extreme pain and then death.

She decided to fight the cancer as long and as hard as she could, and deployed in this battle her great reserves of courage and stoicism. She accepted all the help medicine had to offer – surgery, chemotherapy, radiotherapy, meditation, breathing and mobility exercises. She refused to move to a hospice, and was able to remain at home thanks in large part to the Hampstead District Nursing Service, in particular the support of a wonderfully skilled and sensitive nurse, Sister Sandra Beevor.

At periods, she became very withdrawn – as described in Marilyn Hacker's 'Against Elegies' (page 109). Commenting on one of these moods afterwards, she said that she had seen 'everything and nothing', and that they were the same.

A few weeks after completing a portrait of her dog (in which she made use of the unsteadiness of her hand to get a delicate and strangely spiritual effect) and only two days after completing a long article on machinery for printing business forms, her system collapsed over just a few hours in the night, and she died on the morning of 1 December 1991.

During the months of her illness, Catherine continued with her freelance work and – usually working from about 3 am until dawn – made the charcoal sketches of 'The Cancer Drawings: Another Way of Seeing'. These drawings are visions: they show a world which is real, but invisible – until the veil has been ripped away. The veil is our fantasy that life is a safe, permanent condition ruled by human laws. The world behind it is a place of violence, cruelty and chaos; but it contains love and the possibility of peace, and it is, in its fierce way, beautiful.

Like many visions, these come out of dreams, recollections of childhood, religious and mythological images (themselves visions), sensations of the body, and the search for something which makes sense when the answers provided by our collective consciousness fail to make sense. They are also informed by Catherine's long search for something beyond transience. They express too the weird, mischievous and witty parallels she saw between things. And they tell a story.

The story begins with the discovery of the lump, or the foetus ('The Egg', frontispiece), which glows with the dawning life within it. Consciousness follows ('The Gestation', page xii) as this strange new being changes the outline of its mother as it grows, as if the genes of the foetus were given to the parent rather than the other way around. The third drawing, 'Mother' (page xviii) reflects on Catherine's personal experience – her mother had had breast cancer; her father stomach cancer. Here, a woman, one of her own breasts flaming, suckles her swaddled papoose, in whose tiny breast is the spark of a new flame. Unlike the nervy first two drawings, this one is calm, quiet. The mother, drawn as an Amerindian woodcarving, has the remote solemnity of a deity; her breast is also a hand, held up in priest-like blessing; the only movement is the gentle tug of the infant at the breast.

For Catherine Arthur

The story continues with a narrative of treatment. 'Mrs Beeton's Cow' (page xxvi) follows the good cook's identification of the more succulent parts of the animal; it shows the subject, on hands and knees, marked out into chuck, brisket and so on, in the crudely-drawn lines used to guide the surgeon's knife. In 'Surgery' (page 34), she lies in a vulva-shaped serving dish. Poised, masked and remote above her, the doctors toy with their knives and forks. 'Radiotherapy' (page 52) follows surgery; the simultaneous sensations of burning and freezing that accompany this treatment cause the subject's body to arc out of a flaming sea, as if receiving an electric shock. In 'Chemotherapy' (page 60) she idles in slashed leather and jeans against a wall topped with broken glass. She has a bristling punk haircut (chemotherapy makes your hair fall out), her jacket is sliced and stitched over the breast, and the drug-graffiti on the wall gives the chemical formulae for this intra-venous treatment. These drawings are angry and resentful; the sufferer is isolated; they are also cruelly funny.

The central visions which follow take the series on to another plane, showing the connection between knowledge given by cancer and natural or supernatural forces. Perhaps these could be called the phase of acceptance, of entry into the new state, and contemplation of it. 'Diana' (page 102) (like 'Actaeon's Hound', page 114, taken from Titian) shows the goddess with her bow, her cancerous right breast cut off to free her for shooting. In the quiver lies a baby, the child of the 'Mother' drawing, asleep, trusting. The baby's breast too is mutilated.

The drawing of 'Sedna' (page 134) shows the woman's body (which was taut and muscular in the first drawing, but gradually loses its defin-ition) disintegrating, as Sedna's body did, according to the Inuit myth. Sedna refused to marry the man chosen for her by her father, and he, in revenge, forced her to marry his dogs. Sedna escaped by flinging herself into the waves. Her body broke into the creatures of the sea and fed the people of the Arctic.

In 'Anubis' (page 164) the jackal-headed Egyptian God of the Dead holds the subject in his arms. She is headless (has the jackal eaten her head?) and her breast is a black hole. But Anubis has a protective air as he looks about him. His alert, pricked ears resemble those of Catherine's dog. His breast, too, is cancerous, a vortex of white pain. Look closer and this vortex is also a pool where bathers relax while a small figure dives into the centre. This mysterious tiny figure – the foetus during birth, the hanged man of the Tarot, perhaps an image of sex, or spiritual bondage, or of the willingness to undergo ordeal in a process of birth or rebirth – is a motif in many of Catherine's paintings and drawings.

As the series progresses, images of death become more frequent, and the process more distinctively a rite of passage. In 'Standing Stones' (page 178), the hole in the megalith through which the dawn sun shines is a breast cut out by cancer. In 'Corn Circles' (page 196), the mystery of these strange forms is solved: here they are a fiery force preparing to consume the neatly regimented order of industrial farming, or – since the field is also a woman's body – mechanised living.

In describing 'Boadicea' (page 230), the last of the series, it would be difficult to improve on Amanda Sebestyen's words in a *Feminist Review* article:

> Irony informs Catherine Arthur's most beautiful image of death, 'Boudicca' [*sic*]. A tree carries life forward, fed by the body of a woman. At the same time, the tree is a placenta, nourishing her as a foetus waiting under the earth. The lost breast, inside the skeleton, flowers as a rose. But the tree is exactly the shape of a mushroom cloud.

Though Catherine Arthur, who was always suspicious of grand labels, didn't want these drawings to be seen as art, she did hope that they would be useful to other people facing cancer in its terminal form, and illuminating to those as yet unable to look into the face of death. It would be impertinent to try to sum up in words what has been so magnificently said in images, but perhaps one could hazard one conclusion: that cancer, the black hole, the cruel energy within all life that drives the predator and the prey, the irresistible Other, can also give a terrible freedom – to reject the comfort of fantasy and acknowledge the dark and mysterious forces by which we are possessed.

For Catherine Arthur

AGAINST ELEGIES

Marilyn Hacker
For Catherine Arthur and Melvin Dixon

James has cancer. Catherine has cancer.
Melvin had AIDS.
Whom will I call, and get no answer?
My old friends, my new friends who are old,
or older, sixty, seventy, take pills
with meals or after dinner. Arthritis
scourges them. But irremediable night is
father away from them; they seem to hold
it at bay better than the young-middle-aged
whom something, or another something, kills
before the chapter's finished, the play staged.
The curtains stay down when the light fades.

Morose, unanswerable, the list
of thirty-and forty-year-old suicides
(friends' lovers, friends' daughters) insists
in its lengthening: something's wrong.
The sixty-five-year-olds are splendid, vying
with each other in work hours and wit.
They bring their generosity along,
setting the tone, or not giving a shit.
How well, or how eccentrically, they dress!
Their anecdotes are to the point, or wide
enough to make room for discrepancies.
But their children are dying.

Natalie died by gas in Montpeyroux.
In San Francisco, Ralph died
of lung cancer, AIDS years later, Lew
wrote to me. Lew, who, at forty-five,

expected to be dead of drink, who, ten
years on, wasn't, instead, survived
a gentle, bright, impatient younger man.
(Cliché: he falls in love with younger men.)
Natalie's father came, and Natalie,
as if she never had been there, was gone.
Michèle closes up their house (where she
was born). She shrouded every glass inside

– mirrors, photographs – with sheets, as Jews
do, though she's not a Jew.
James knows, he thinks, as much as he wants to.
He hasn't seen a doctor since November.
They made the diagnosis in July.
Catherine is back in radiotherapy.
Her schoolboy haircut, prematurely gray,
now frames a face aging with other numbers:
'stage two,' 'stage three' mean more than 'fifty-one'
and mean, precisely, nothing, which is why
she stares at nothing: lawn chair, stone,
bird, leaf; brusquely turns off the news.

I hope they will be sixty in ten years
and know I used their names
as flares in a polluted atmosphere,
as private reasons where reason obtains
no quarter. Children in the streets
still die in grandfathers' good wars.
Pregnant women with AIDS, schoolgirls, crack whores,
die faster than men do, in more pain,
are more likely than men to die alone.
And our statistics, on the day I meet
the lump in my breast, you phone
the doctor to see if your test results came?

For Catherine Arthur

The earth-black woman in the bed beside
Lidia on the AIDS floor – deaf, and blind:
I want to know if, no, how, she died.
The husband, who'd stopped visiting, returned?
He brought the little boy, those nursery-
school smiles taped on the walls? She traced
her name on Lidia's face
when one of them needed something. She learned
some Braille that week. Most of the time, she slept.
Nobody knew the baby's HIV
status. Sleeping, awake, she wept.
And I left her name behind.

And Lidia, where's she
who got her act so clean
of rum and Salem Filters and cocaine
after her passing husband passed it on?
As soon as she knew
she phoned and told her mother she had AIDS
but no, she wouldn't come back to San Juan.
Sipping *cafe con leche* with dessert,
in a blue robe, thick hair in braids,
she beamed: her life was on the right
track, now. But the cysts hurt
too much to sleep through the night.

No one was promised a shapely life
ending in a tutelary vision.
No one was promised: if
you're a genuinely irreplaceable
grandmother or editor
you will not need to be replaced.
When I die, the death I face
will more than likely be illogical:

Alzheimer's or a milk truck: the absurd.
The Talmud teaches we become impure
when we die, profane dirt, once the word
that spoke this life in us had been withdrawn,

the letter taken from the envelope.
If we believe the letter will be read,
some curiosity, some hope
come with knowing that we die.
But this was another century
in which we made death humanly obscene:
Soweto El Salvador Kurdistan
Armenia Shatila Baghdad Hanoi
Auschwitz Each one, unique as our lives are,
taints what's left with complicity,
makes everyone living a survivor
who will, or won't bear witness for the dead.

I can only bear witness for my own
dead and dying, whom I've often failed:
unanswered letters, unattempted phone
calls, against these fictions. A fiction winds
her watch in sunlight, cancer ticking bone
to shards. A fiction looks
at proofs of a too-hastily finished book
that may be published before he goes blind.
The old, who tell good stories, half expect
that what's written in their chromosomes
will come true, that history won't interject
a virus or a siren or a sealed
train to where age is irrelevant.
The old rebbetzin at Ravensbrück
died in the most wrong place, at the wrong time.
What do the young know different?

For Catherine Arthur

No partisans are waiting in the woods
to welcome them. Siblings who stayed home
count down doom. Revolution became
a dinner party in a fast-food chain,
a vendetta for an abscessed crime,
a hard-on market for consumer goods.
A living man reads a dead woman's book.
She wrote it; then, he knows, she was turned in.

For every partisan
there are a million gratuitous
deaths from hunger, all-American
mass murders, small wars,
the old diseases and the new.
Who dies well? The privilege
of asking doesn't have to do with age.
For most of us
no question what our deaths, our lives, mean.
At the end, Catherine will know what she knew,
and James will, and Melvin,
and I, in no one's stories, as we are.

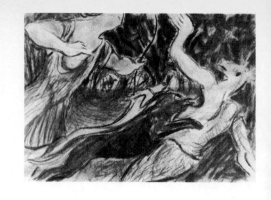

Actaeon's Hound

Refugees in a Strange Country
Carole Colbourn

Shock and panic, like cancer itself, spread silently and unseen. The effects can become apparent suddenly and unexpectedly. The damage may be beyond limitation or the situation may be retrieved and life will go on. But life goes on changed.

This story, written jointly by a husband and wife, is about a GP with a young family who discovered she had breast cancer late in 1989. It tells of her own feelings over the following six years and the reverberations of the trauma for the people close to her.

Phil

I felt something unusual. I suppose I said something to Carole, who felt it and looked a bit troubled. I could guess what might be going through her mind. It's not the sort of thing you want to talk about. It hangs in the air, an unvoiced fear, an unspoken anxiety. 'I don't suppose it's anything important.' What one of us said, both of us hoped. 'I suppose I'd better go and have it checked.'

Carole

I dutifully went to my GP. I knew what the statistics were. At 39 I had a 90 per cent chance that it would be benign. But why did it feel so irregular? It is interesting that my husband found it. I expect that so-called 'self-discovery' usually means 'partner'.

Only a few weeks earlier I had referred back to the hospital a patient with a recurrent breast cancer. It had been treated in the first place only with excision, a lumpectomy, followed by a course of the drug Tamoxifen. As it turned out, this had been a totally inadequate treatment. I remember she had two daughters still at school.

I showed the report to our senior partner. He had seen her when the problem had first arisen. 'I'm glad I don't have breasts,' he said.

When I was a medical student in London we had studied with a famous breast surgeon. We had seen things on the ward that I could still remember with a mixture of dread and horror. I could think of no worse disease or condition. Twenty-five years ago there was heroic surgery in the form of 'radical mastectomy'. This involved removing the muscle under the breast. Oestrogens are thought to play a part in at least some breast cancers, so if there was a recurrence the hormone supply was cut off by removing the ovaries. In some cases the gland sited in the brain that controls ovary function, among other things – the pituitary – was removed. I can remember seeing women in the later stages of the disease, lying emaciated and helpless on their beds, immobilized by the pain.

My GP referred me to the local hospital. The surgeon examined me and said he would have to take some cells with a needle to check the pathology. He said he would refer me for a mammogram. As he filled in the form for the referral, he read the letter from my GP again. 'I'm sorry,' he said, looking up, 'I didn't know who you were.' In other words he had just realised I was a GP. But there was still not much communication or support. It wasn't that I expected special consideration, more dismay that this was the standard treatment. Since I knew the general statistics and the difficulty of predicting an outcome for an individual, it seemed pointless to ask too many questions. Later, when

I returned for the test results, he said simply, 'It's cancer, and you know as well as I do what that means.'

One night when I was on call soon after receiving the bad news I sat up until 3am in the surgery flat leafing through whatever books and information I could find. I decided not to take any of it home. It is always more difficult to tell other people the realistic odds: this is one of the problems GPs constantly have to grapple with. We try to dwell on the hope present in a situation and only when it is apparent that treatment is failing do we confront people with the tough realities of terminal illness. I now knew that with no node involvement, the chances of my surviving another ten years were perhaps six out of ten. In general cancer terms this is quite good. In personal terms it was a disaster. It was not a good idea to share this knowledge with my family.

I had been back in general practice for only a year. I had taken 10 years out for the children, doing baby clinics and school medicals to keep my hand in. The children were now 11, 10 and 7, the youngest a girl. It had always been my ambition to be a principal in general practice. My partners responded with shock. 'How awful!' 'You *have* got a problem.' 'Cancel all your surgeries, now, for as long as you need.' My Mum said, 'Why isn't it me?' On a later occasion she referred to the fact that I am a Christian. 'You have your faith,' she said. It was true, but if my future depended on my feeble effort at faith, I didn't stand much of a chance. If God was there, he would have to sort it out by himself. There was not much we could do, except hold his hand and hope. We dared not look much into the future.

The local hospital did not have a specialist cancer team.

At a second interview, this time with my husband present, the surgeon asked if I wanted a mastectomy. Well, what did he *think*? In fact, it was the only treatment on offer. As far as I was concerned, I had breastfed three children and I was not expecting any more, so I could afford to lose one. But Phil might feel differently.

I found the lack of personal support at the hospital distressing. I don't remember one doctor or nurse who lingered long enough to ask how I was feeling or to find out how I was coping emotionally. I wasn't sure if people were avoiding me because I was 'the doctor'. The physio-therapist let me cry and I was grateful for that. She said, 'I know. You want to see your grandchildren.' I had already worked out that the chances of seeing my daughter through school were less than 50 per cent. I resolved that I would teach her the things I had not spent enough time on until now – cooking, sewing, knitting. 'Please, God, I do not want my daughter growing into adulthood without her Mum.'

After the operation, the surgeon said, 'Oh, you'll be all right.' It had a hollow ring. He said he would ask another doctor at the hospital who took an interest in cancer and chemotherapy to see me. It was not very clear what programme of treatment he meant me to have; after that he went on holiday. When I saw his second-in-command he said that he must have meant me to see a visiting specialist from a hospital many miles away, about radiotherapy. He did not think chemotherapy was appropriate and was confident I should have radiotherapy to the chest area. 'There are no nodes involved,' he told me. 'All chemotherapy will do is blast your ovaries. I might as well do that with radiotherapy.' (Was that supposed to be a joke?)

The radiotherapy raised difficult questions. Where? It was at least 80 miles to the nearest centre: should I travel there and back five days a week for five weeks or more? It did not sound like a good idea. Should I stay in a hostel at the hospital with other women undergoing the same treatment? The prospect was completely depressing.

In the end I asked to be referred to a hospital in the city where I grew up. At least then I could stay with my Mum, and Phil and the boys could carry on at home as normal. His parents went over to help out and friends rallied round. I took my daughter with me: she stayed with my sister for six weeks, going to school with her cousin, who is the same age. Mum and I both felt awkward about talking so we buried our anxieties in decorating her kitchen. My parents are divorced. My father knew about the operation but did not contact me and I did not contact him. He still lived in my home city, but I had no desire to discuss these things with his new wife.

But this was some weeks away. First there was Christmas.

When I went to the hospital for the results of the initial tests, they did an X-ray and then asked me to come back in an hour to speak to the surgeon. I knew something must be wrong. What can you do for an hour while you wait for your death sentence? I went shopping. I plunged into the town, in the shops, round the market, buying Christmas presents for the children. Christmas was coming. At this rate it could be my last. Damn! Damn! Damn!

What do I want for Christmas? Pretty obvious; but on second thoughts, I decided that I would like an eternity ring. My engagement ring had always been awkward for everyday use; an eternity ring would be more practical and, of course, eternal. It signified that I intended to be around for a long time and that we wanted to be together. Spending a lot of money on the ring was like taking out insurance on the future.

The boys didn't say much. John wanted to know if having the operation meant it was something serious. 'Well,' I said, 'quite serious but I'll be fine afterwards.' How much do you tell them? Robert had just started at secondary school. I was horrified at the school biology he came home with: the common causes of death – cancer, including breast cancer. I hoped he hadn't guessed.

The operation was over. No one felt like doing the preparations for Christmas so we booked Christmas dinner at a local hotel. It was unnerving, being jolly with a load of strangers. I stuffed a pair of tights into my bra to fill it out. The children had never seen bright blue sorbet before. Neither had we. It was a landmark on our journey. We were refugees in a strange country.

Phil

It was all a bit of a whirlwind. You just had to do what you had to do. Did I want my wife to have a breast cut off? No, of course not. But did I want my wife to die? You just had to hope that despite all the doubt and confusion the decisions you made would be the right ones. You had no way of knowing.

You want to do something practical. I latched on to the idea of moving house. If we could move into town we would be nearer the hospital. Then if the worst came to the worst, we would all be near at hand. In retrospect it sounds like defeatist talk. At the time I would have said it was being realistic. But Carole could not face the thought of moving, so we put it aside.

Talk to someone. Yes, of course, I needed to talk to someone. But most of my friends were patients of the group of GPs my wife worked with, and she didn't want everyone in town to know. We were attending a local Methodist church at the time and they had what they called 'pastoral visitors', each responsible for part of the congregation. Jan, our PV, was the wife of a good friend. She came to see me while Carole was in hospital for the mastectomy, and gave me the opportunity to voice my fears. I was always struggling to keep back the tears around that time, I seem to remember. Typical man! (Trying to keep them back, I mean.) After that I seemed just to carry on. Writing down scraps of thoughts as poems was my only outlet.

While Carole was away for the radiotherapy I learned a lot about housekeeping and childcare. I discovered that after you think you have done everything there are always still three more things to do. Every night I allowed myself to go to bed only when I thought I had got it down to three, and only three, outstanding jobs. The anxieties got buried under the practicalities. Keep busy; don't try to think.

Carole

The problems were building all the time beneath the surface. While I was away for radiotherapy we couldn't talk very well on the phone and the weekend visits were no better. We dealt with the day-to-day things, living one day at a time, and tried to get our sense of what was important into a new order. But we suppressed much of our anxiety and most of our real needs.

I had some good friends who would hold my hand and cry with me. Friends often apologised that they were not much help, but the sharing of tears and fears was the best thing they could have given me. I still could not bring myself to share the statistical facts that were underlying my fears. I didn't think it would help anyone, either them or me.

As I was returning to work the government was busy changing the rules. The new GP contract came into force in 1990. I had started as a part-time GP – it was all I wanted to do with my responsibilities for a growing family. But overnight the terms were changed and I could not continue to work the hours I had chosen. The contract insisted that I work five days a week as well as nights and weekends on call, with no time off in lieu. The workload on call was a no-win situation: if I chose to spend the night at the practice flat there would be no calls; if I decided to go home there would be three, nicely spaced out so I reached home each time before being called out again. In some ways it was easier to stay at the flat. I rationalized it to myself: it was good for Phil and the children to learn to cope without me, just in case the worst happened.

Life became more and more frantic. Phil and I passed like ships in the night. I wanted to cut my hours, but there did not seem to be any way to do it without making life difficult for my partners at the practice. And I could not leave and start again somewhere else because I was no longer a good employment risk. Eventually we hit on the idea of job sharing, and a likely looking 'other-half' was found by one of my partner GPs. I am glad to say that she has become a good friend as well as my other-half partner at work. But the hours have gone on creeping up and up. I still do not have the time to do all the things with my daughter that I said I was going to do. She is now 13.

It was terrible going back to work after four months away, but I was too morbid to stay at home. I needed something to occupy my mind and some social contact – we were living in a beautiful place but it was way out of town and too far away from friends. But I soon realised that I had changed. All the trivial things people came in with made me cross. I was now completely intolerant of people moaning about aches and pains, especially if they were getting on in years. What did they expect? They should be grateful to be alive! What right had they to be upset at their mortality?

I went back to visit the patient with advancing breast cancer. She had had a year of treatment which resulted in some improvement, but eventually a steady decline set in. I had to be there. I needed to see what actually happened. She received very good care and treatment; she had high doses of painkillers; she was comfortable. It was better than it had been 25 years before.

Gradually I learned to talk to patients going through the crisis of cancer, especially younger women with breast or cervical cancers. I have shared my own history with many of them. Often they say that there is no one else with whom they can talk. One said she did not want all the staff where she works to know. She said she read the stories of publicity in the papers about well-known women and their fight against breast cancer and wondered if her reaction was peculiar. I told her I felt exactly the same way. It still alarms me that sometimes other people feel free to share my story.

I try to put my patients' problems in perspective when I talk to them. If there is some life-threatening illness then I know that now I can relate to it better. Not all patients want to talk. Some find it difficult, especially men. I do not probe. I try to ask them to come back for another appointment, and often on a second visit they will admit what is on their mind. Frequently I spend a long time with a patient, much more than the allocated 5–10 minutes. I think it is probably more useful than a lot of the other jobs I am asked to do. But there are still times when I get it wrong and put my foot in it.

My cancer provoked a mid-life crisis, especially for my husband. What is this phenomenon? If life begins at 40, perhaps it is adolescence. Critical life experiences occur, you are running low on energy, the children are pushing back the boundaries, elderly parents become a source of worry. Perhaps it is not surprising that someone panics. Marriages crack, people commit suicide, resort to alcohol and make irrational decisions. We stared into the abyss and teetered on the edge. We forget that life is change, that it is possible to adapt to altered circumstances. But sometimes it is necessary to retreat before we can regroup and re-enter the lines.

Two years on and I was functioning more normally. At that time there was a lot of coverage of a big trial of breast cancer treatments in the

Lancet. There was a growing trend for using chemotherapy to treat younger women; the idea was that it would mop up any stray 'seeds' of the cancer that might be floating round the body. I had not had any chemo. Should I have had some?

I plucked up courage to go to my GP and ask her if she could refer me to a cancer specialist. She arranged an appointment at the Royal Marsden Hospital in London. Then I began to feel awkward: was I using my position 'in the trade' to gain an unfair advantage? I justified it to myself by reasoning that talking to a specialist would help me answer my own patients' questions when they came to me with their worries.

I had asked, when I had the operation, if they could grade the tumour. How serious was it? Could they measure if it was especially sensitive to oestrogens? I had been told that this was done only for research purposes. The specialist in London asked to see the history of my tumour. Luckily the local hospital still had a microscope slide of it, which they sent to him. He had it visually graded: apparently it was a fairly serious type, middle grade. He would have advised chemotherapy had he seen me at the time of my operation. As it was, I had been lucky. I was still here and well. I didn't know whether to be relieved, grateful, or angry.

The specialist recommended that I should start on Tamoxifen. He reckoned that it should be recommended to all breast-cancer patients. The radiotherapist had also suggested that I could take Tamoxifen, though he said that its effectiveness is not proven in pre-menopausal women. Tamoxifen is an anti-oestrogen and taking it could exacerbate any menopausal tendency. I did not want an early menopause, thank you very much, but I decided to give it a go. The Tamoxifen question – should I or shouldn't I, what will happen if I do and what will happen if I don't? – is still unresolved six years later.

I started on a standard dose. All of a sudden I seemed to be upsetting everyone – the staff at work, the patients, the family at home. The family would definitely not tolerate much more of this: I was proving very difficult to live with. I stopped taking the Tamoxifen. I had to talk to someone, so I saw a specialist who assured me that my reaction was quite common: the brand of the drug I was taking was a cheap version imported from Eastern Europe, and some people experienced a bad response to it. The original brand, made by ICI in the UK, had less severe side-effects. I got it changed.

Unfortunately my troubles were not over. There was no doubt that I was less grumpy and irascible, and my husband was talking to me again. But now I developed a troublesome dryness of the vagina and lost interest in sex. Talking was all very well, but not enough to keep my husband happy for ever. Whatever I did with this stuff, he seemed to be losing out. I could not discuss the Tamoxifen question rationally with him. All he would say was, 'How do I know?' I wanted him to say yes or no: either he could do without sex or he couldn't. I needed to make a decision.

I talked the situation over with some of my female colleagues and stopped taking Tamoxifen, again. Do you take a treatment that is supposed to increase your life expectancy or do you opt for quality of life? If the treatment is very likely to help you might be prepared to put up with the side-effects, but if you believe it is likely to make only a small difference then any side-effects weigh more heavily in the balance. Life is to be lived now. I didn't want to take something that will affect the quality of my life for the rest of my days. Better a livable life now, however brief, than a prolonged miserable existence. Quality of life was becoming increasingly important to me.

It was not until two years later that I started Tamoxifen again. This time it was a smaller dose and I had the use of an oestrogen cream to counteract the vaginal dryness. I arrived at this compromise after talking to a specialist at our 'local' Breast Centre (actually 80 miles away) where I now go for follow-up and regular check-ups. Looking back at my experience of treatment by the local hospital I now understood what my patients were having to go through. But none of us knew any better at the time. We are the last outpost in a rural area; the National Breast Screening Service did not reach us until summer 1993. Then we discovered the existence of the specialist breast clinics. Until that point we had not been properly informed about what was available, and we were GPs.

As we found out more, our pattern of referral changed. Woman who went to the Breast Centre came back full of praise for the efficient and caring approach, and were happy to go back for follow-up. We started to send more people. But this caused some friction with the local hospital, which depended on us for their work and the money that went with it. From their point of view, 'breasts were their bread and butter'.

We had a meeting with them. One of our partners was trying to negotiate for improvements in the service. 'You have to come too,' she said to me. 'I can't say anything,' I protested. 'Well you'll just have to tell me what to say.' I jotted down some notes from the MacMillan Breast Cancer leaflet and went along. We sat across the table from the hospital team. I dug her in the ribs whenever I thought there was something that needed to be said. At one point one of the surgeons commented, 'What's so special about breasts anyway?' At the time there was no way I could have given an answer that was fit to be heard in public. Here is a more reasoned response to why breasts – and specialist care for them – matter.

Answer 1. Ask any straight man. If he was being honest he would tell you it is a stupid question.

Answer 2. Breast cancer kills children's mothers. It is the most frequent cancer to affect women in the UK. One woman in 12 will develop a breast cancer at some time in her life, and it is the prime cause of death for young women in the age range 35–49. Three of my friends at university, as young teenagers, had lost their mothers to breast cancer.

Answer 3. Britain has one of the highest incidences of breast cancer in the world, and one of the highest death rates. Are we so badly organized that we cannot do anything to change this? I suspect that had it been men who suffered from this condition it would have been given a higher priority.

Answer 4. We do not know what causes breast cancer. There are not many other major killers about which we are so ignorant. Research may help. There has recently been news of a breast cancer gene that could be used to identify which of those women with close relatives who have breast cancer are themselves high-risk.

Answer 5. Mastectomy is surely the most frequently performed mutilating procedure carried out in British hospitals. It has a drastic effect on a woman's body image. It has drastic effects on those women's partners, too.

Answer 6. The type of treatment affects the length of survival for many women, even though cure is not possible. This buys valuable years.

As GPs we are very encouraged by the recent government-led initiative to establish Cancer Centres, centres of excellence, in all regions of the UK. The stated aim is that specialists should work together to establish protocols for the treatment and management of cancer patients. There are well-organised services for screening family members in the US, but here in the UK it is haphazard. The specialist cancer units are gradually giving guidance more generally, but in the meantime the reaction of a general surgical unit or of a non-involved GP is likely to be, 'If your sister is the one with the problem, why do I need to see *you*?'

For me, the chief difficulties after the operation were the practical ones. I did not feel comfortable going swimming anymore, though I am more than happy just to sit in the jacuzzi – it feels like an indulgence and I need a reward for daring to change in the public changing room. I have never dressed revealingly, so I did not particularly mourn my cleavage. But there have been times when my new state has caused me embarrassment, especially if I find myself out on call with clothes thrown over my nightwear that fail to make good my deficiency.

Obviously I was worried about physical rejection by Phil. At first I clung to him: I desperately needed the physical affirmation that I was still here, and that he knew I was still there. Gradually we busied ourselves with the day-to-day jobs and I began to feel that I was withdrawing. Was it my imagination or was Phil avoiding looking at me? I worried about losing him: nobody else would take me on in my reduced condition.

I am a practical sort of person and it is my job to be practical about bodies. Both Phil and I tend to be undemonstrative: neither of us had ever felt particularly free to express ourselves physically. As a result, perhaps, we were becoming physically and emotionally distanced from each other as the years went on. It does tend to happen anyway, I think. After several years with children in the bed it is not surprising. You go to bed worn out and you get up worn out. Things are so busy with a first baby that I used to wonder how anyone ever got the time to make another one. But things were beginning to improve as the children got older and less intrusive. I can remember thinking that we would have to wait until the children had left home for the chance to be fully expressive in our relationship. Then the operation came and sent everything back to the dark ages.

After the operation I began to realise that I didn't even get much chance to look at myself. We had no lock on the bedroom door, and the bathroom mirror didn't reveal much. At last we read in a book the advice to put a lock on the bedroom door. It was the start of a new era. We could now begin the long slow process of learning to accept each other again. Why it had never occurred to us before I shall never know: what a shame that it was only now, after I had been mutilated by the operation, that we began to find a new openness. How much better if we had done it when I could have been proud to be whole. If you have children, and if they are invading your space, put a lock on the bedroom door *now*.

Phil had to learn to accept me, but that could only come after I had learned to accept myself. I needed confidence. Only then could we begin to come close to each other emotionally and physically. Only then could we learn again to express ourselves through the body freely. But my confidence was to be shattered first.

Marriages are apt to flounder. It is not surprising. Who is inadequate? It is easy to get negative and defensive and to feel threatened. The threats are real. I implored God not to let it happen to me. I did not want our marriage to break up.

Phil

Perhaps I need to say something from my point of view here. I will try to be honest. Without doubt, women have an effect on me. I like nothing better than to see a pretty face, for example. But I am a committed Christian and I believe in the importance and necessity of marriage. We have been made this way: the husband needs the wife and the wife needs the husband. And I don't think it would be putting it too strongly to say that I need my wife's breasts. They are essential to my emotional well-being. An attack on my wife's breasts is an attack on me. It undermines my emotional stability.

It is only now, having survived to year six, that I can begin to recognise how I really felt. At the time, of course, we both coped with the situation the best we could. 'Oh course I don't mind you only having one breast.' I am sure I must have said it, probably more than once. 'You are more important to me than a breast.' 'What's so important about a breast?' I might have added. Of course I meant it and believed it at the time. But I was fooling myself and denying the strength of my feelings.

I am sure that I thought that Carole needed strong support from me rather than a binge of self-pity, that the last thing she would want would be for me to be constantly drawing attention to what, for her, must have been a worse loss. On reflection I was probably wrong. She tells me that as far as she was concerned her breasts could be cut off. They had done their job. They had fed three babies. So, in point of fact I was the only one who needed them. But I would not have liked to have admitted this to anyone, not even my wife.

I had not the insight to realise that I had gone through the same crisis before, after the birth of our first child. Being deprived of free access to my wife I was tempted to think of alternatives, though fortunately it was only in the mind. Now I was jealous of other people who had, or had access to, what I imagined were a perfect pair.

It took three or four years and the death of my mother to crack me, but in the end crack me it did. I found myself signed off work for six weeks and signed on to anti-depressants. I had fallen into an infatuation. We had the roughest period of our relationship. Carole said that if that was the way I was thinking, then we had to do something serious to save our marriage. That frightened me thoroughly. I felt as though I was staring down the barrels of a double-barrelled shotgun. I was only human, I reasoned, and I felt completely trapped in my situation. We were held together for a time only by the slender thread of our shared view of marriage.

Some friends, recognising that we were having a crisis of some sort, suggested that we see the minister of our church. I don't think I was too keen at the time, but in the end we made an appointment. It did not get better overnight, but from then on we were putting solid ground back underneath our feet. There was still an evening when I fled round to the minister's house in a panic and on the verge of tears. There were still times when it seemed hopeless. I met with the minister and another friend from the church regularly for many months. Old traits of character had to be dug out and the ground made good with a new understanding of God's love. I learned to see the word 'repentence' in a new light, discovering that it was a positive, not a negative thing. It was the way into creation, making everything new, a fresh start. In the end our weekly meeting over lunch became a mutual support group. The other two have now both moved away, but there are still links of a special, human kind.

Those two men and my wife helped to haul me out of the pit. I am very grateful to them. As a result our marriage has grown stronger: more intimate, more real, more supportive. Nothing is perfect and nothing stays the same, but we now know more about ourselves than we did, and we know more about each other. We also know that forgiveness is the heart of it. From that grows strength.

Carole

It was now 1993: year three. We were preparing to move house at last. Against the run of the housing market and despite losing our original purchaser we had stitched up a three-cornered deal. We were going down the hill nearer to civilisation. It would be warmer, drier and free of midges.

Phil's mother had been ill and died in the New Year. Nobody would say what the initial cause of her dramatic decline was, but it was certainly a spreading cancer and could well have been breast cancer. Did they really not know or where they just not saying?

We lived over 200 miles away and had not been close in recent years. The children experienced their first funeral but, as it was a cremation, there is no place where Grandma can be 'visited'. It has made me think about how we end our time on earth. I have decided that I must think of a suitable place where those who are still here can go to to remember me.

We were busy with sorting and packing. My arms seemed to feel heavy and my left arm was definitely getting swollen. I had had a left-side mastectomy: you can imagine the sinking feeling. What was going on? Was this …? Back to my GP, who diagnosed a simple phlebitis. Rest was the prescription; that impossible thing. But could it be something more sinister?

It was at Easter that Phil admitted that he was having problems; we moved in May. The rest of the year was a very rough ride indeed. Just after we moved some friends told us of the death from breast cancer of a mutual friend. Our friends reported that she had died in peace, ready to go, a wonderful death. I panicked. 'I'm not bloody dying nicely!' I told Phil later. I definitely was not ready to go to heaven, however good it might be, or anywhere else for that matter. I had better things to do down here.

I went into work each day feeling insecure. I usually rang Phil during the day or he rang me. We both needed reassurance. I cried with my partner at work on many occasions. I would tell her that I could not cope if I had to lose the other breast. I was convinced that it would mean the end of my marriage, and beyond that it would be downhill all the way. I was becoming irrational.

I needed to let go. I had to let Phil go and not imprison him; to trust that he and God together would work it out. And I needed to let go of the children in the sense that I had to trust God to look after them if anything happened to me. I loved them. I had to believe that He loved them too.

I still need to learn to let go. I have made a start. In the Gospels, Jesus says that if you would gain your life you must lose it. I am beginning to understand. When He tells us to deny ourselves He is only reminding us that this is what He does. God does not demand our love. He waits for us. He is happy when we come freely to love. It is the same with our human relationships.

It is all bound up with me letting go of my own life; losing it. I know I have a long way to go before I achieve this attitude fully, but this beginning to understand has helped me with some of my worries.

It occurs to me that letting go is what I have had to learn to do, as far as my patients are concerned, ever since I qualified as a doctor. I cannot be personally responsible for the behaviour of all my patients. All I can do is to be there, alongside, as a fellow human being, ready to help if and when I can. Each one of us has the ultimate responsibility for ourselves. Everyone has to make their own decisions before God. It is not up to me.

Meanwhile, I prevailed on everyone to get me referred to a specialist cancer centre 80 miles away. Nothing else would satisfy me. The doctor there understood my panic and gave me the whole works. Everything came out clear. The bone-scan was the first I had had for three years. I should have had one before, he informed me. At last I felt that someone was prepared to take me seriously. I began to calm down.

One possibility that I began to consider seriously at about this time was breast reconstruction. One of my female partners at the practice had strongly urged me to think about this at the start, but we had rejected her advice. Now I was beginning to find that in some situations the prosthesis was a problem. I could not always keep myself together. At a Barn Dance I would feel myself coming apart in the middle of a dance, usually when progressing towards some young stranger. Things did improve when I got a new prosthesis (apparently I should have gone to get one sooner; they didn't tell us about these things at Medical School). At a post-graduate lecture, a professor of surgery mentioned breast reconstruction using the spare tyre from the tummy, tissue from the abdominal flap. Great idea! It would get rid of my extra tummy at the same time.

I tried to gauge Phil's reaction. He seemed non-committal. In the end we decided that reconstruction would result in yet another physical change that we would have to adjust to. Having got close to each other after four years adrift I don't want to risk another disruption. It is something that needs to be considered soon after the mastectomy, if there is a chance. At the time, though, the decisions seem too many and too awesome.

Phil

Coming to terms with Carole's survival seems to have been more of a problem than coping with the prospect of her imminent death. In a sense I had already grieved for Carole – in the months after the first discovery I went through much of the process of bereavement. I had to sort out in my own mind how I was going to cope should the worst come to the worst. Recognising that she was still going to be around but that life had changed required a different kind of adjustment.

Carole

We keep on having to review our situation, rethink our priorities. The children are growing up quickly. They will soon be leaving home. We still have not told them specifically about it all, though they know we have had problems.

I try to think what I can do to lessen the risk to my daughter. There is nothing conclusive in the literature I have read. I try to ensure that we have a healthy lifestyle: we don't smoke, we limit alcohol to a reasonable minimum, we eat fruit and vegetables and have cut down on dairy fat. I try to take more exercise.

We have cut non-essential activities outside the home to a minimum. Phil stopped going to conferences and meetings away from home, and tries to fit what he does around my work schedule. We have to find a way of ordering things so that we can all function properly.

There are things we try to make time for. Time for exercise, to cycle or walk. Time to talk, to see friends, to unburden the stresses of the day or the week. Time to be thankful for the day.

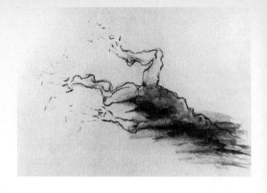

Sedna

The Lump
Evelyn Dale

I was diagnosed as suffering from breast cancer in 1989. I was a 20-year-old undergraduate at Oxford University. There was no history of breast cancer in my family, I had never taken the Pill and had rarely smoked. The diagnosis seemed totally inexplicable and incomprehensible: all I could think was, 'why me?' I still had a residual belief from my childhood that I was immortal. Breast cancer brought me in touch with my mortality.

As part of trying to come to terms with my diagnosis I scoured reference books to find the physical or emotional causes of the illness, trying to come up with a rational explanation. But many of the theories did not apply to me, while in other cases the books and articles contradicted each other. As well as physical causes I wanted to know about psychological factors. Some books seemed to suggest that the disease was linked with certain personality types – for instance, women who repress their feelings, especially guilt or anger. For a short time I frantically 'psycho-analysed' myself to see if my personality matched that of the sufferers described.

As a teenager I had always been slightly obsessive, especially about my schoolwork and appearance. I had demanded a great deal of myself academically, often working until late at night and yet still feeling that I had not done the work meticulously enough. Although my weight was normal for my height, I used to attend as many aerobics classes as I could, supplemented by a vigorous hour-long workout every evening. I also used to swim regularly and walk every day. As a result of my reading about breast cancer I began to feel guilty, wondering whether through my obsessive hard work and exercise I was directly responsible for causing my illness. I began to feel that my personality might be to blame. Gradually, as I started my course of treatment and became more confident in my recovery, I succeeded in weaning myself off my dependency on reading about the illness and could place the theories in perspective. I realised that my reading was in part an attempt to reassure myself that I would get better – that the cancer would never return.

As a child I had heard only about people who had died of cancer, never those who had made a full recovery. As a result cancer for me evoked the torture of a series of painful treatments involving high doses of radiotherapy or drugs with unpleasant side-effects which would finally prove ineffective. Making changes in my perceptions of cancer played an important role in helping me to cope with my diagnosis. I realised that cancer was not necessarily a death sentence, and came to see it as a potentially enriching, rather than negative, experience.

I first became aware that there was something wrong in August 1988. While on holiday after I had finished my 'A' levels, I started to experience a 'pinprick' sensation in my left breast. The feeling lasted only a couple of days, and once it had disappeared I forgot all about it. Then a week after I started at university, the morning of the matriculation ceremony, I woke up feeling tired and unwell: I had a bad cold and I started to experience the same 'pinprick' sensation again. But since the pain was only intermittent, I did not see the point in seeing a doctor. I never even thought of examining my breasts (before Sixth Form College I had attended a Roman Catholic school, where health-related issues were studiously avoided). About two weeks later, while I was writing an essay in my room, I felt a sharp spasm of pain shoot through my breast. This time the pain was intense, like a hot needle puncturing the skin. Alarmed, I started to feel my breast. Just below the areola I found a small, hard lump. Instinctively I knew at once that I had cancer.

I started to remember all the people I had known who had died of cancer. I was terrified of dying, especially at the age of 20. I was a creature of habit and routine: I liked to get up at the same time each morning and adhere to the work timetable I had drawn up. Any disruption, however minor, worried me. Now, as a result of my discovery, my life would be in a state of disarray. Any treatment would result in my neatly planned days having to be completely re-arranged, and I couldn't bear the thought of sitting in hospital waiting rooms while everybody else got on with their lives. There was no time in my life for illness, so I decided not to spare the lump a second thought and to carry on as though nothing had happened.

But ignoring the breast lump was not as easy as I had imagined. During menstruation the pain in my breast would be almost unbearable, and I had to take painkillers to try to control it. Often I would lie down and wait for the waves of pain to subside. At night, in bed, I would touch the lump to see whether I could detect any changes, always hoping it might have disappeared. But it was always there, always the same – small, solid and immovable. It felt like a hard dried pea.

I imagined a chaotic, haphazard arrangement of cells that had clustered together to form a tumour. I sometimes wondered whether a 'corrupted' cell might be brushed away from the others as I touched the lump, floating away to adhere to vital organs, causing them to become cancerous too. So far nobody knew about the cancer except me. There were no visible signs that I had the illness. Sometimes I wondered if I would die if I ignored the lump, and how long this would take. I imagined being told by an oncologist that the lump had been detected too late and that there was nothing anyone could do to help me. But although the thought of dying terrified me, I still could not bring myself to seek medical help. I did not want my suspicions that I had cancer confirmed.

Gradually I managed to persuade myself that the lump could not possibly be malignant but was just a swollen gland or mastitis. 'Women aged 20 simply don't get breast cancer,' I assured myself. 'It's completely unheard of.' As I had no other symptoms associated with cancer, I convinced myself there could be nothing seriously wrong.

Just before Christmas 1988, home for the vacation, I made an appointment to see a doctor near my parents' house. I had been suffering from a sore throat which never seemed to clear up. While I was telling the doctor about my throat, I briefly considered mentioning the lump but decided not to as I thought that she would most likely simply dismiss it as nothing to worry about and make me feel silly. For the next few weeks my throat was constantly sore and I felt tired and run down. I went to the doctor's surgery several times, was prescribed several courses of antibiotics and had blood tests for anaemia and glandular fever. Every time I went to the surgery I wanted to be able to tell the doctor about the lump, but I never felt able to do so.

My first reaction when I found the lump had been one of deep shock. This sense of shock was gradually replaced by a numbness so great that it prevented me from thinking logically or rationally, blotting out my awareness of the fact that the sooner treatment for cancer is commenced, the less likely the cancer is to spread. I was paralysed by terror: at the age of 20, my greatest fear was of having a mastectomy, irrespective of whether or not the operation would save my life. I also delayed seeing a doctor because I needed to adjust to the idea that my life would be changed dramatically by the illness. I needed to come to terms with the fact that I had cancer before I could tell anyone about it. At last I gained sufficient strength to feel able to face going to hospital and undergoing treatment. I finally accepted that the lump was not going to disappear of its own accord, and that if I did not seek medical help, I might die.

Two days before I was due to return to college I told my mother in a matter-of-fact way that I had discovered a lump in my left breast. She looked alarmed, telling me that any abnormality should always be treated seriously. She told me to make an appointment to see a doctor as quickly as possible. Since the beginning of the spring term was imminent, I agreed to see one of the doctors at college.

But it was not until the pain started to come back that I at last went to the surgery to see the college nurse. By this time I had also noticed that I was unable to move my left arm properly – it often hurt to stretch it forwards or upwards. The nurse listened sympathetically and told me I was probably suffering from mastitis. She made an appointment for me to see one of the college doctors that afternoon. I felt better immediately, partly because the burden of carrying the 'secret' for so long had been lifted and partly because I was confident that the lump would be diagnosed and treated quickly. However, this visit heralded the beginning of a three-month battle with doctors before my self-diagnosis of breast cancer was confirmed.

'I have a small lump in my left breast. It's beginning to worry me because it's been there for nearly three months and it doesn't show any signs of going away or getting smaller.' I spoke tentatively because I felt embarrassed about the apparently trivial nature of my complaint – I did not dare to suggest I thought I might have cancer. The doctor was very brusque. 'Well, I doubt very much that it's anything serious. It's probably just a cyst. Young women are prone to these. Still, I'll examine it.' He proceeded to examine each breast carefully. After the examination, he told me that he could not find a lump at all. I was stunned. 'There is a lump there,' I insisted, pointing to the place where I had felt it. My fears that I might not be treated seriously had been confirmed, and I felt confused and humiliated. The doctor examined my left breast again. 'I can assure you,' he repeated, 'there's absolutely nothing there. All women experience tender, lumpy breasts at one time or another. But if you're complaining of breast pain, I'll prescribe you some diuretics which should help ease it.' He asked me to make another appointment to see him after I had completed the course of tablets if the symptoms had not disappeared. Although I felt sceptical about the benefits of taking the diuretics, the hope that the lump might just be a swelling which would respond to the tablets did not quite disappear.

I swallowed the diuretics dutifully, regularly checking my breast, hoping that the lump would vanish. But it remained exactly the same size and as hard and immovable as ever. After a fortnight had elapsed I made another appointment to see the college doctor. I explained that I was certain that I could still feel a lump in my breast, but this time he refused even to examine me, telling me that I was not to make another appointment to see him about this particular 'problem'. He started to ask me how I was settling into university, trying to find out whether I was depressed.

For several weeks I vacillated between forgetting the lump and making an appointment to see another doctor. There were times when I wondered whether the lump really was just a figment of my imagination, but the increasing pain and the difficulty I experienced when stretching my arm were enough to remind me that something was wrong. By the end of February 1989, almost six weeks after I had last seen the college doctor, the pain was becoming unbearable. I decided to take a break from college and go home for a few days. I made an appointment with the doctor whom I had seen during the Christmas vacation.

'The lump is nothing to worry about at all,' the doctor assured me after she had examined my left breast. She explained that it was just a fibroadenoma or benign tumour, and told me to make another appointment to see her when I came home again at the beginning of the Easter vacation. She would decide then whether or not the lump ought to be removed. A tremendous wave of relief swept over me. I did have a breast lump, but it was not malignant. For a little while I was convinced that I had not got cancer after all.

In late March I made another appointment to see the same doctor. By now my feelings of relief at her diagnosis were starting to be replaced by the old nagging doubt. How could she be sure that the lump was not malignant if no biopsy had been performed? I decided to ask to see a surgeon; an appointment was made for three weeks' time. This seemed like an eternity, though I tried to keep busy so I would not have too much time to brood. I saw the surgeon in April, six months after I had discovered the lump. While I was sitting in the waiting room I wondered whether this would be the day when at last I would find out whether or not I had cancer.

After the surgeon examined my breast, he told me the lump was a benign tumour. He said that my inability to move my arm properly was not related to the lump in any way, though later I was to discover that difficulty in moving the arm on the side of the affected breast is one of the signs that a lump may be malignant. No biopsy was offered. I asked him if he could make arrangements for the lump to be removed – although it was not visible, I found the idea of its presence disfiguring. He agreed but warned me that I would have to wait another two weeks. Despite his certainty that the lump was harmless I had a sense of time running out. I was terrified of the cancer spreading while I battled in vain to be taken seriously.

I was admitted to hospital for the removal of the lump on 13 April. Everyone had assured me that the lump was benign, but I still felt frightened and unsure. When I came around from the operation I felt very tense and the pain in my breast was excruciating. Despite the assurance that I had received that I did not have cancer and that, even if I did, they would not perform a mastectomy without consulting me, I was distressed at the idea that my breast might have been removed without my knowledge. I was taken back to my room, where the nurses pulled down the blinds in silence and left. Suddenly I felt very alone. My drowsiness started to wear off and was replaced by an over-whelming nausea, exacerbated by my anxiety. I was convinced that something was wrong. Later my mother came to visit and told me that an appointment had been made to see the surgeon again the following Monday. The surgeon had told me that no follow-up treatment would be necessary, so the fact that he had recalled me alarmed me. I longed for somebody to explain what was happening, but nothing was said.

My mind began to work overtime. I began to wonder whether something had gone wrong during the operation itself. The possibilities seemed endless. I had a raging headache, I was very hot and my sides hurt from the repeated bouts of vomiting. I was sure that one of the reasons I felt so ill was my worry about what was going on, but the nurses seemed to become uncomfortable as soon as I began to ask any questions.

For several hours I slept lightly. When I woke up I felt exhausted, but at least the nausea had disappeared. It was a beautiful spring day and I began to feel more confident. But my panic returned as soon as I saw the expression on the surgeon's face as he walked into my room. 'Did the operation go well?' I asked nervously. 'Was the lump just a benign tumour?' I desperately wanted him to give me some definite answers. But he remained infuriatingly non-committal, telling me I'd have to wait until Monday when he'd see me at his clinic and give me the test results. Suddenly I felt angry, sensing that I was being kept in the dark. Several months later I discovered that the surgeon had in fact warned my mother and sister that I might have breast cancer even before he visited me.

I was desperate to return home as quickly as possible. While I was packing my suitcase I kept thinking about the test results. I felt as though I had been concussed – everything seemed blurred and indistinct. I kept wondering what would happen if I had cancer and whether I was going to die. I was terrified.

Just before I left one of the nurses came to see me. 'I know that you're worried about the diagnosis but it's important not to get too disheartened at this stage. And even if the worst comes to the worst and you have got cancer, there are many things that can be done to help you.' 'Is is always necessary to have a mastectomy?' I asked. 'No. Sometimes the lump alone can be removed, which means that the breast can be preserved.' She told me a story about a young boy she knew who had been given chemotherapy for bone cancer and had made a full recovery. I began to feel slightly better.

Nervous energy helped me to survive the weekend. But though I kept myself as busy as possible, I thought about the lump constantly. I was too anxious to sleep and I began to dread going to bed because my thoughts would inevitably turn to the cancer. I longed for the waiting to be over, and literally counted the hours until I was due to see the surgeon again.

By Monday morning I felt a fresh surge of optimism. 'Statistically, only one lump in every 10 proves to be malignant,' I assured myself. Over the weekend I had reasoned that the surgeon would not have made an appointment for me to see him so quickly unless he thought that the lump was serious. But while I was in the waiting room I began to hope for a 'reprieve'.

The surgeon was sitting at a table in a heavily-blinded room. His hands were folded on the desk. I immediately felt uneasy. 'I'm afraid…' he began awkwardly. 'I'm afraid that the news isn't very good. The breast lump was small but it was malignant. I've arranged for you to have a body scan at the department of nuclear medicine on Wednesday morning at 9 o'clock. I've also made an appointment for you to see an oncologist on Friday morning. By this time, he'll have had a chance to look at the results of your body scan and to determine whether the breast lump is a primary or a secondary tumour. At the moment we cannot tell whether the cancer has spread to the lymph nodes and whether other organs are affected too.'

The news was broken very quickly – within the space of a couple of minutes. I remained silent, trying to absorb its impact, trying to think of something to say. I wanted to tell him that everyone had assured me that there was no possibility that I had cancer, so how could the tests be accurate? I wanted to ask him why I had had to wait for so long just to have my own suspicions confirmed. I had forgotten all the questions I had prepared. I froze. 'The oncologist will arrange for you to have a liver ultrasound to see whether the cancer has spread to the liver,' he continued. 'You'll have to start a course of radiotherapy but I'm not sure what other treatment he will decide on. You certainly shouldn't be thinking of returning to college this term. The radiotherapy and the visits to the hospital will take up too much time and your treatment should be given priority.' 'Can I have some sleeping tablets?' I asked suddenly. 'I can't sleep any more, even though I feel so tired.' I felt disorientated and unable to think of anything else to say. 'Yes,' he replied briskly. 'Make an appointment to see your doctor tomorrow and she'll prescribe some.'

I had reached the point where I was so frightened my mind was blocking things out. I felt as though I was in a dream – everything seemed more vivid than usual and the events that were unfolding had no sense of reality. I rang the people who had asked to be told the results of the tests and informed them that the lump had been malignant, but I was scarcely able to believe that I was talking about myself. I wrote letters to my tutors at college explaining that I would be unable to return for the summer term. I was anxious about falling behind in my work and dreaded the prospect that I might not be allowed to go back to college at all.

By Wednesday, the day of the body scan, I felt more positive about the diagnosis. I felt like a ball which has been squashed and slowly starts to revert to its normal shape. The following day I was taken out by my cousin, which helped to distract my thoughts. A bouquet of flowers arrived from some of my friends at college, along with sympathetic and encouraging letters from my tutors. These helped to elevate my mood. Most of the time I felt too blurry to think about the impending results of the scan, but occasionally I would panic. I imagined being told that the cancer had spread everywhere and that nothing could be done for me. Every twinge of pain I experienced terrified me. At other times I imagined being telephoned by the hospital and told that a mistake had been made and that I had been given the wrong results.

'I'm pleased to tell you that the scan was clear, which is very encouraging.' The oncologist's tone was gentle and reassuring. I began to feel more optimistic as he spoke. 'I'm sure it must be a great relief for you,' he continued. 'At least the uncertainty is now over. The breast tumour is a primary tumour. I'll still arrange for you to have a liver ultrasound, although I'm confident that it'll be negative. Perhaps you would like to ask me some questions before we start discussing your treatment.'

'Will I have to have a mastectomy?' I asked. At the age of 20 I could think of nothing worse. 'No,' he replied. 'The tumour was small and I believe that a lumpectomy combined with radiotherapy is the best option.' All the other questions I desperately wanted to ask and had carefully rehearsed poured out – what are the chances of a recurrence, what caused the tumour to grow, what can I do to prevent a recurrence? The oncologist's replies were always considered and careful; he never committed himself to an answer. At first I found it difficult to deal with the lack of certainty – I still had a child's need for definite answers. But as time progressed I came to terms with his inability to predict an outcome, and stopped seeking 'omniscience' from him.

I felt more optimistic after I had seen the oncologist. My appetite improved and I started to reduce the number of sleeping tablets I was taking. He had recommended that I begin my treatment with radiotherapy and about 10 days later, after my scar had had a chance to heal, I returned to the hospital to be 'marked'. By this time I had received all the results of the remaining tests, including the liver ultrasound, which confirmed that the cancer had not spread. The radiographer took me to a side room and proceeded to draw a series of lines in erasable ink on my shoulders and ribcage to show where the beam was to be directed. 'Do you mind if I give you two small black tattoos?' The thought of tattoos on my body which would serve as reminders of my treatment upset me, but she reassured me that they would just be two tiny dots which would gradually fade.

'I'm afraid that you won't be able to have a proper bath or shower while you're having radiotherapy,' she continued. 'If you get the skin on your back and shoulders wet it will cause the lines to fade, but more importantly the area being treated and the skin surrounding it can become sore and inflamed and may react badly to soap and water or to anti-perspirant.' My heart sank. The weather was almost unbearably hot and there were to be times during the treatment when I longed for nothing more than a cool shower or a long, relaxing bath, especially when I felt tired and nauseated. During this time I went through a phase of scouring self-help books to discover methods or preventing a recurrence. I experimented with different diets and herbal teas, but in the end opted simply for a well-balanced diet, especially since I often felt unwell while I was having treatment.

I remember having walked past the radiotherapy unit at the hospital a few times when I was a child. The place had seemed eerie and isolated and the warning signs about the danger of radiation conjured up images of Hiroshima. My childhood impressions were hardly softened when I started to receive treatment there. The unit consisted of a network of dark corridors decorated with a few pictures made up of shapes including capsule-like cylinders, circles and crosses whose haphazard arrangement reminded me of cancer cells. The treatment room itself made me think of the interior of a submarine. There was a single 'port-hole' through which the radiographers could observe the patient and control the treatment by pressing a panel of buttons. Once I was on the table the radiographers went out of the room, switching off the lights and leaving me alone and isolated.

I continued to receive radiotherapy three times a week throughout May. A friend would always accompany me to the hospital, which made the visits more bearable, especially as it was not unusual to have to wait for several hours before being seen. Sometimes I felt very unwell after the treatment and I experienced a persistent feeling of nausea which meant that I ate very little. Milk-based drinks were my staple diet. But the side-effects subsided once the treatment stopped. The mobility of my left arm was excellent after the operation and the breast healed rapidly. The livid bruising soon disappeared completely, and a scarcely perceptible, silvery pink line where the incision had been made was the only trace of the operation.

One of the most distressing aspects of my treatment was seeing very young cancer patients and those whose lives seemed dominated completely by an uncontrollable disease. As a child I had believed that I was immune from ageing and death. Particularly when I saw children suffering from the disease, I was reminded of the fragility of human life and of our helplessness and limitations.

On my way to see the oncologist for check-ups I used to pass the recovery room for patients who were receiving chemotherapy. I remember seeing them clutching ice packs to their scalps to minimise the hair loss, or curled up like embryos in their beds, their lives seem-ingly dependent on their bodies' tolerance of the powerful drugs in the small bags of colourless fluid attached to drip stands. 'I've discussed your treatment with an oncologist at the Royal Marsden Hospital and we feel that it's best for you to have chemotherapy after you've finished your course of radiotherapy,' the oncologist told me towards the end of the month. I had almost forgotten that chemotherapy might be a possibility and had begun to believe that my ordeal would soon be over and that I could forget about cancer altogether. I felt the same cold terror I had experienced when I was waiting in the surgeon's clinic only six weeks earlier to find out whether I had cancer. I dreaded the prospect of chemotherapy: drugs which attacked cancer cells by poisoning the entire body seemed a primitive, crude and haphazard method of treatment. For a moment I felt angry with myself and again blamed myself for my illness. I felt defiled by the disease and totally helpless. A wave of despair swept over me – the first time I had experienced such a feeling since the news that I had cancer had been broken to me.

'Will I lose all my hair?' I asked suddenly. I hated the idea of being physically disfigured by the drugs. 'No, I think that's extremely unlikely. You'll probably notice thinning rather than total hair loss,' the oncologist replied. 'Does the treatment make all patients vomit and feel unwell?' I persisted. 'If you feel nauseous, I can prescribe some anti-sickness drugs,' he offered. 'When you are given chemotherapy drugs intravenously I'll make sure that you're given anti-sickness drugs intravenously at the same time. This should help to minimise any unpleasant side-effects.' For a few seconds I contemplated committing suicide if things become intolerable. This seemed my only method of showing that I still had some control over my life, and I derived some comfort from the thought. I was concerned not only about losing my hair but about feeling tired and nauseated for several more months. I longed to have a healthy appetite and resented having to go to bed in the afternoons to rest. The treatment also made me feel isolated: I missed the social life at college and found it difficult to talk to my friends about what I was going through, since their own experience of 'serious' illness was confined to glandular fever. 'It's ironic that I felt so much better before I had the operation and started the treatment than afterwards,' I thought. But as time passed the prospect of chemotherapy started to seem a challenge and gave me a greater impetus to fight the illness.

My treatment began in early June. I was to be given a triple 'cocktail' of drugs – Fluorcil, Methotrexate and Cyclophosphamide. The Fluorcil and Methotrexate were to be given intravenously on two consecutive Fridays each month; in the 14 days in between I would take Cyclophosphamide tablets orally. The two-week interlude between finishing one course of tablets and injections and starting another would give the healthy cells a chance to recover. The treatment would be given over a period of three to six months, depending on how well I responded.

After my first injections I collected my prescriptions for anti-emetics and Cyclophosphamide at the outpatients' clinic and drove to the town centre to have lunch and do some shopping. I was surprised at how quickly the injections could be administered compared with the length of time needed for radiotherapy. I felt liberated from the burden of having to attend the hospital three times a week and I was able to study and read in my new-found spare time. I started to establish a routine – I would get up fairly late to maximise my rest and would fill up the rest of the day with walks and college work. Towards the end of June my friends came down from university for the summer vacations and I stopped feeling so insular and began to dwell less on the cancer since I was able to go out more.

Just before I had started my course at university the previous October I had booked a holiday to California with my mother and brother. During the months of treatment, I looked forward constantly to this holiday and it gave me an incentive to carry on. While I was on holiday I began to feel less tired emotionally and was glad to have a respite from hospitals and medical treatment. I relaxed on the beach, though I had to wear a T-shirt to protect the area which had been treated during radiotherapy. I started to notice that when I washed my hair there were more hairs left in the shower than usual, but large clumps were not falling out.

The new term at college was due to begin in October and I was feeling apprehensive about returning, combined with a longing to get back to normal life and put the 'cancer chapter' behind me. I wondered whether I would be able to cope with the demands of the work, though I had tried to keep up as much as I could during my term off. I was still undergoing chemotherapy treatment and it was not long before I realised that the time taken up by my visits to the hospital meant that I had to work unreasonably hard in the intervals. I noticed larger amounts of hair clogging the basin and more strands of it in my hairbrush. I began to feel under intense pressure. I was terrified of admitting defeat, though I was pushing myself to breaking point, against the oncologist's advice. In the end I decided to see my tutor about the possibility of reducing my workload. It was agreed that instead of taking 12 papers that spring, I would only have to take four, but I would be able to pass provided that these were of a satisfactory standard. My anxiety decreased and I no longer felt guilty about sleeping for a couple of hours in the afternoons. My hair loss also started to diminish.

My moods tended to ricochet at this time: sometimes I felt able to cope, but at others I felt extremely unsettled. This was not helped by the fact that I was spending half my life at home recuperating after treatment and the other half at college. Before I had cancer I had felt in control of my life and had trusted in my ability to do things. But the cancer was eroding my confidence, especially since I often blamed myself for the illness. Now I found myself with self-doubt and frequently felt inadequate compared with the rest of my peer group. But the illness also had compensations; I noticed that the things that worried other students, such as examinations and finding jobs after they graduated, did not trouble me to the same extent. My priorities had changed rapidly, with good health at the top of the list. I also started to find reserves of inner strength when confronted with difficult situations.

I continued to receive chemotherapy throughout the autumn term. One of the side-effects was a feeling of lethargy which produced a craving for sweet things. I ate vast amounts of chocolate, starchy puddings and biscuits and my weight soared from 7st 11lb to 9st 6lb. I became too self-conscious to wear jeans and dressed in skirts instead. The drugs made my hair look lank so I usually wore it scraped back into a chignon. I felt ashamed to go to the hairdresser in case he noticed that my hair was thinner and questioned me about it. I suddenly felt older, and this was reflected in my appearance. But as soon as the treatment was over I lost the excess weight, had my hair cut and started to wear casual clothing again.

I had three sessions of chemotherapy. At times those months seemed like an eternity. Sometimes I felt I couldn't face any more of it and I had to force myself to go to hospital for the injections. I hated the side-effects – tiredness, nausea, lethargy – and longed to finish the treatment because I believed it would symbolise the end of the illness and I would be able to erase the cancer from my mind. It would be as though nothing had happened.

I tried to imagine I was swallowing little 'kalashnikovs' each time I took the Cyclophosphamide. I visualised the tablets as 'guns' that would kill the enemy cells which were invading my body. I imagined two warring factions: the unhealthy cancer cells versus my healthy cells reinforced by the chemotherapy drugs fighting on their side. But as in any war there were casualties. Healthy cells were sometimes innocent victims caught in the crossfire and had to die alongside the enemy. My body outwardly 'mourned' the loss of its allies with fatigue and nausea.

I finished my treatment in December 1989, 14 months after my initial discovery of the tumour. I had carefully discussed the advantages and disadvantages of continuing the chemotherapy with the oncologist, and decided to call a halt since there was no guarantee that my chances of a full recovery would be any greater after six or nine courses. I felt an overwhelming sense of relief when the treatment ended. It was as though a cease-fire had been declared on my body. I was grateful for a suspension of the battle.

My life for several months afterwards was a period of readjustment. Initially I thought I would be able to snap back into my old routine; I expected to come through the experience unscathed; I thought I could blot out the cancer from my consciousness. For some time I tried unsuccessfully to battle against the memories – I loathed spending any time thinking or talking about the cancer and hated dredging up the past, especially the painful memories of the weekend I had spent waiting to find out whether or not I had cancer. But after a while I came to terms with what had happened and accepted that I had been ill with a potentially life-threatening disease. I tried to see the positive aspects of the illness rather than dwelling on the negative ones, and this became the touchstone of my ability to survive.

The fear of a recurrence haunted me. Sometimes I would have nightmares that I was dying from cancer, which would cast a shadow over the following day. If I experienced a spasm of pain in my back I became convinced I was suffering from cancer of the spine. If I saw a bruise I would be sure I had developed leukaemia. I rigorously checked my breasts, anticipating that at any moment I might discover a large tumour. The passage of time helped to heal some of my anxiety and I became able to distinguish between health vigilance and neurotic obsessiveness. Although the nausea wore off after I stopped taking the drugs, I continued to feel tired for several months.

Since I had had a lumpectomy rather than a mastectomy I did not have to cope with the loss of a breast. I did, however, have to come to terms with the appearance of my left breast following the operation. For about a year the tissue surrounding the area where the lump had been removed remained hard, as though cardboard had been inserted subcutaneously. The breast also shrank slightly, making it difficult to buy underwear that fitted well since the left breast was almost one cup size smaller than the right. Sometimes I felt depressed at the crumpled appearance of my bra on the left side – there were creases which were conspicuous under certain types of clothing. I experimented with different makes of bra until I found a type which fitted almost perfectly. This helped to increase my self-confidence.

Sometimes I felt the cancer had undermined my femininity and after the treatment I started to spend a great deal of money on clothes, cosmetics and accessories to compensate. I sought constant reassurance that I was still attractive and lived in constant fear of rejection. I felt as though I was 'shop-soiled goods' in comparison with other members of my peer group.

My attitude towards the cancer varied. Sometimes I was able to rationalise what had happened – I reminded myself that everyone's life is at risk on a day-to-day basis and no one knows for certain when they will die. But at other times it was as if a sword of Damocles was hanging above my head, ready to fall at any moment. I felt confused by the disease and my anxiety gnawed away at me insidiously. I constantly doubted myself and started to feel I was incapable of achieving anything – that I had failed and let other people down.

These emotions were tempered by a tremendous sense of optimism and gratitude that I was still alive. As a result of the illness everything in the world seemed to have been painted with a brighter, richer palette; everything seemed sharper and more clearly focused. Time suddenly became very precious and I longed to cram as much into each day as I could. I resisted the temptation of saying that I had had a bad day, knowing that the day could never be repeated. I tried to live for the moment and avoided planning ahead, fully aware of life's unpre-dictability.

Initially I had check-ups every three months. I asked for blood tests at regular intervals to check for abnormalities; I had an annual bone scan. After two years had elapsed my outpatient appointments were reduced to once every six months. In 1994 the oncologist asked me whether I would like to discontinue these appointments because five years had elapsed, but I preferred to continue to see him on a six-monthly basis for the sake of my peace of mind. I finished my degree course in June 1992 and started to train to be a teacher in September 1993. After I qualified I accepted a teaching post at a school in London.

Just after the autumn term began I succumbed to tonsillitis and laryngitis but refused to take any time off to recover. A few weeks later I started to experience tenderness under my right arm. I made an appointment to see a doctor, who said he thought the pain was most likely to be the result of a strained tendon. He prescribed an anti-inflammatory cream and told me that if the symptoms did not improve after a week, I was to come back. Although the symptoms cleared up quickly I still had a nagging feeling that something was wrong.

About a fortnight later I experienced a stabbing pain in my left arm and breast. I persuaded myself that it was only pre-menstrual breast tenderness, but the pain reminded me of my symptoms of six years before. I felt frightened, but the next day the pain had almost gone. I heaved a sigh of relief and put my fears to the back of my mind. Only a few days later, however, I was having a bath when I accidentally hit my rib cage underneath my left arm. A sharp spasm of pain passed through it. I had hit a small lump. For a few seconds, everything went black. I sat up in the water and kept on feeling this lump. Surely I was mistaken. There was probably something similar on the other side. I felt my right armpit frantically but there was nothing there. Just this small, hard lump on the left side.

'There is a swollen lymph node under the left arm, but they're swollen under the right arm too,' the oncologist said reassuringly when I saw him the following day. I don't think they're cancerous – it's possible that you cut yourself when you were shaving the armpit, which might have caused the lymph nodes to become swollen. For the time being, we'll blame the razor, but I'll check them again in a fortnight's time.' I left the hospital feeling almost jubilant, but my sense of relief was transient. Deep down I was starting to experience the same nagging doubts I had had before. During the two-week interlude I did not dare touch my rib cage in case the lump was still there. I was frightened of confirming my own fears.

'Yes. That node is still there, though the glands under the right arm have completely disappeared. We need to discuss this.' I was panic-stricken. 'Is it cancer?' I finally forced myself to ask. 'I'm not sure,' he replied cautiously. 'I would say there's a 50 per cent chance that it is. I'll contact a surgeon and ask him to remove it as soon as possible.' He carried on speaking for a while, but I was too dazed to take in what he said and have hardly any recollection of it.

I left the hospital and went home in a state of confusion. Everything I had rebuilt so painstakingly over the past five years seemed to have been swept away within the space of 20 minutes. It was though I had just watched a wave wash over a sand castle. Finally the surgeon, whom I had last seen five and a half years before, telephoned. He said he would be able to perform the operation in two days' time, on Thursday. I asked him how long I would have to wait to receive the results; he told me he would be able to give me them the same afternoon.

For the next 48 hours I felt as though I was re-living the nightmare of my past. I hardly slept at all the first night, and when I woke up the following morning I felt depressed and hopeless. The next day I drove to the hospital. I was filled with memories of going to the same hospital five years previously. Everything looked exactly the same. I even wondered whether I would have the same room I had been given last time.

Though the surgeon had been optimistic before the operation, I knew as soon as I saw his expression when he came to see me afterwards that something was wrong. He gently explained that the node was cancerous, but that I had not suffered a recurrence of the disease. A cell from the original tumour had been lodged in one of the lymph nodes and had slowly developed into a small tumour over the past five years. As a result of the anaesthetic, I felt too numb to understand fully what he was telling me. I remember experiencing an acute sense of disappointment suffused with sadness before I fell back to sleep again.

The oncologist visited me the following morning. He explained again the nature of the lump and how he was planning to treat it. I would not be given radiotherapy this time – six months of chemotherapy seemed the most appropriate treatment. He told me he wanted me to have a bone scan and a liver ultrasound, though he was almost certain these would be clear. I sat on the bed trying to absorb the impact of what had happened. I felt as though I was falling down a long, smooth-sided tunnel; I could not cling to the sides and there was no light at the end of it. After he left I started to pack my suitcase, waiting for my mother to collect me as I had done five years before. It was the day before Christmas Eve.

I dreaded the prospect of returning to school after the holidays, terrified in case I would break down in front of a class, but in fact I was surprised by how quickly I was able to get back into a work routine. Teaching classes helped to divert my attention from the cancer and the prospect of chemotherapy, though sometimes I was guiltily aware of feeling almost envious of the children, remembering my own adolescence when I too had been healthy. I was always conscious of having to retain my composure and never allow my anxiety to show. Though I sometimes found it difficult to get up in the mornings because I felt tired, once I arrived at school I was busy and energetic. But as soon as I came home again my energy would evaporate. Sometimes I would slump on the sofa and be unable to get up for hours, overcome by lethargy. 'I feel like a puppet,' I once explained to a friend. 'During the day, somebody pulls the strings and I function automatically. But in the evening when I'm alone I am floppy and lifeless.' Usually I would fall asleep from mental exhaustion at about 8 pm. One Saturday afternoon I drove to a nearby shopping centre and, after I had parked, had to rest for half an hour in the car.

The thought of a second bout of chemotherapy distressed me. At first I felt too depressed and tired to ask the oncologist whether there was any alternative, and passively accepted that I would begin six months of treatment as soon as I had finished my teaching contract at the end of February. But I did not want to do it. I kept remembering that chemotherapy carried the risk of inducing an early menopause. One evening I became so anxious about this that I rang the oncologist to ask him whether this was likely. He told me that, while the drugs often made older women menopausal, he was uncertain what would happen to me. But he admitted that since I had already had chemotherapy five years earlier, the risk with a second bout of treatment would be greater.

I hated the idea of being menopausal at the age of 26. I imagined my hair becoming thinner, I imagined developing osteoporosis. I felt everyone had turned against me and became almost convinced that they wanted me to undergo the treatment in a deliberate attempt to maim me. My depression and lethargy gave way to anger and renewed energy. This time *I* was going to choose my treatment. One evening I told my parents that I was not going to have chemotherapy. I had made up my mind that I wanted to have further surgery to remove the rest of the lymph nodes under my left arm. I also wanted to try hormone treatment to get rid of the cancer.

I applied for a place on a journalism course which started in April, leaving a six-week gap between finishing my job and starting my course in which to have the operation. I also decided that, before I ruled out chemotherapy, I would seek a second opinion. My oncologist agreed to make an appointment for me to see another oncologist at the Royal Marsden Hospital.

'After reading the letter which your oncologist has sent me,' he began, 'I feel that chemotherapy is the most appropriate form of treatment for you.' I listened patiently. I had come to the hospital with an open mind. I had not expected him to suggest hormone treatment, but I refused to allow myself to be put off asking for the treatment I wanted. Part of my resistance to chemotherapy stemmed from a feeling that I was being 'pushed' into it: it was as though the consultant had a mental picture of a set of data – which treatments had the greatest success rates for particular age groups – and I had not been considered as an individual or had my wishes taken into account. I glanced at the oncologist for a second. 'It's not *your* internal organs and health which are going to be damaged by chemotherapy,' I thought. I remembered the friend who had advised me to seek a second opinion: 'It's your life,' she had said.

So I embarked on an explanation of my reservations about chemotherapy. 'I have a very bad gynaecological history,' I added. 'Is there any possibility that the cancer may be hormonally linked?' He paused for a few minutes. 'I was unaware of these difficulties, since they were not included in your letter of referral,' he said. 'As your cancer is slow growing, there is a possibility that it may be a hormonal cancer. Perhaps you would like to try Tamoxifen instead of chemotherapy?' He explained that Tamoxifen is a hormonal drug and gave me a brief outline of how it works. He also suggested that the lymph nodes under my left arm should be removed, to help reduce the risk of cancer in the future.

I felt as though a huge weight had been lifted from my shoulders. I would not have to endure six months of painful injections, nausea and

constant tiredness. In addition, I made an appointment to see a gynae-
cologist who was interested in possible links between diet and
hormonal abnormalities. He put me on a strict diet of starchy snacks at
three-hourly intervals. Within a short time I began to experience fewer
pre-menstrual symptoms that I normally did. A combination of the
new diet, Tamoxifen and Evening Primrose oil capsules eradicated my
breast tenderness.

In early March I saw the surgeon who was going to remove my
lymph nodes. 'It's very important that you are encouraged by the fact
that the cancer has taken such a long time to re-emerge,' he told me.
'It's obviously a very slow-growing tumour.' But I felt anxious.
Although I had had no side-effects from the Tamoxifen to date, I had
read about complications arising after lymph-node removal including
lymphoedema, or swelling of the arm. I was worried that my arm
might become puffy and disfigured after the operation. I took my
customary list of questions from my bag and reeled them off. The
surgeon told me that, while I might experience mild lymphoedema, it
was very unlikely that it would be severe. He suggested that I could
visit the lymphoedema clinic at the Royal Marsden Hospital if I was
worried.

'Before you have the operation, I think it's important that you have
an ultrasound to check that there are no tumours in the right breast
either,' he continued. 'If there are, these can be removed at the same
time.' He explained that an ultrasound was capable of detecting very
small tumours, and said that he would arrange for me to have one the
following day. I started to flounder. 'But I've already got a medical
appointment tomorrow,' I pleaded. 'I might not have enough time to do
both.' I knew that I was playing for time. I did not want to know
whether there were any tumours in the right breast. 'I know you're
worried,' he continued gently, 'but it is very important that any
problems are sorted out at this stage.' Reluctantly, I agreed to go to
hospital the next day.

The results of the ultrasound were normal and the surgeon told me I
would be admitted to the Lister Hospital at the beginning of April.

During this time I began to feel increasingly lethargic. Although I would set my alarm clock for 8 am, usually I would switch it off and sleep until 10 am. Even simple jobs like doing the washing up and making telephone calls exhausted me, and I seemed to spend most of the day lying curled up on the sofa asleep. At first I wondered whether the Tamoxifen was making me tired, but gradually I realised that I was mentally, not physically, exhausted. My feelings of apprehension about the operation were taking their toll. As I walked up the hospital steps I can remember telling myself, 'This is the beginning of the end. Soon I will be able to close this unpleasant chapter in my life.'

When I came round from the operation I noticed that a tube had been stitched underneath my left arm to drain fluid from the wound. The arm was puffy and it ached. I winced at the crumpled appearance of the wound, feeling nauseous and tired. The surgeon visited me the following morning. As soon as I saw him, I knew he had found something. But he was not prepared to discuss it. 'You'll get the tests back on Wednesday or Thursday,' he said. It was now Sunday. After he left I began to sob uncontrollably. Eventually, one of the ward sisters came to reassure me. I told her that I was frightened that if any cancerous cells were found, I would have to have chemotherapy. But she said that no one would stop me from taking Tamoxifen. 'After all,' she added, 'the choice of treatment has to be your decision.' I started to feel better.

On Wednesday the surgeon did not arrive at my bedside until 10 pm, only to tell me that my results were not back yet. In the past, I would have been frantic with worry; this time I hardly cared – I had already steeled myself to accept that there would be some cancerous cells in the lymph nodes. When the surgeon came into the room the following evening, his first words were, 'I think we need to have a chat about your test results, Evelyn.' My heart sank. What was I going to be told this time? 'When I removed your lymph nodes I found 11 of them, and seven of them contained cancerous cells.' My face was expressionless. I was used to it. 'The cancer which we found was left over from last time – from six years ago,' the surgeon continued. 'There is no evidence of any new tumours.' 'What about chemotherapy?' I asked. 'Will I have to have it again?' I was beginning to feel desperate. 'I don't know,' he replied. 'You need to discuss this with your oncologist. But I think that it's very important that you have the treatment you want.'

After he had left I was filled with anger. Why hadn't they taken out the lymph nodes six years ago? Why did I have to re-live this nightmare? On the suggestion of a nurse, the friend who was visiting took me out for a walk. The weather was glorious. As I walked out of the hospital, I felt a sense of disbelief. How could I have lived for six years with seven tumours growing inside me? They had been there all that time and I had never known. We managed to find a café and I talked over my anxieties about chemotherapy, how I was sure that I wanted to keep taking Tamoxifen. 'I did not want to have chemotherapy last time,' I explained, 'but since I was only 20 at the time I didn't dare to question their judgement. Now I have decided that I want to carry on taking Tamoxifen.' I started to feel more positive.

We walked back to the hospital. My friend left and I decided to take a bath. I glanced at the wound again. Even cleaning its surface with a medicated swab nauseated me. I caught sight of my reflection in the mirror as I stepped into the bath. Suddenly I was filled with self-loathing and a sense of self-betrayal. How could my own body have harboured cancer for six years? How could the tumours have failed completely to respond to the chemotherapy? I wanted to be in control. I wanted my body to have been able to get rid of the cancer. But I had failed. I felt humiliated.

I decided to take a sleeping tablet before I went to bed. I drifted off to sleep, waking intermittently. The pain in my arm was excruciating. At one point I walked across to the window. Outside, miles of illuminated London was stretched out beneath me. For a split second I was tempted to jump, wanting to end the misery and uncertainty. Then I noticed that there was the roof of another building directly beneath my window; if I were to jump I would probably only be badly injured. I smiled wryly. My decision had been made for me. I could not kill myself if I wanted to.

I spent most of Friday morning crying. My face became swollen and my eyes were raw. I sobbed, remembering how healthy I had once been, wishing that the lymph nodes had been removed six years ago, feeling frightened and confused. A friend visited me after lunch and we walked down to Sloane Square. It was a beautiful warm April day. I kept remembering that it was almost six years to the day that I had had my first operation.

Once I left hospital I found adjusting to life at home more difficult than I had imagined – at first it was exhausting just to have a bath and wash my hair. My arm felt raw with pain and I took painkillers constantly, counting off the hours until I could take my next dose. Three days after I had been discharged I took my arm out of its sling. At first it felt stiff and detached from the rest of my body, but I was determined to recover its mobility so I tackled the exercises I had been given immediately. Gradually I started to need the painkillers less frequently and I began to feel less tired. My ability to stretch my arm out improved slowly and I was able to go swimming. The arm became less puffy and waterlogged, and the scar began to heal and flatten.

Two weeks after I had been discharged I went back to see the surgeon. He was pleased with my progress and with the appearance of the scar. 'Have you talked to the oncologist about whether you should start chemotherapy or can continue taking Tamoxifen?' he asked. I felt myself turn cold. I had not contacted the oncologist since I had had the operation. I was terrified that he would tell me that I should have chemotherapy straight away, and did not want to be reminded of the large number of lymph nodes involved. Suddenly I became stubborn. 'Look,' I said almost petulantly, 'I do not want to have chemotherapy. It won't work. I want to carry on taking Tamoxifen. I'm due to see the oncologist at the beginning of June and I don't feel that I need to contact him before then.' 'All right,' the surgeon replied. 'I'm not going to argue with you.' Inside I felt a small sense of triumph – triumph at being in control.

Except I was not in control. Deep down I did not feel comfortable with my decision not to discuss the results with the oncologist for another few weeks and not to check whether I should continue to take Tamoxifen. I forced myself to ring him when I got home. He was reassuring. 'Since you are happy with your treatment and you seem to be benefiting from it, I think that you should continue with it,' he said. Suddenly I felt an overwhelming sense of relief. I wished that I had had the courage to ring him sooner to put my mind at rest.

My perceptions of the disease began to change at this time. Six years earlier I had seen the illness as affecting only my breast rather than as a warning from my body to change how I looked after it. But now I wanted to adopt a more holistic approach – to visualise the cancer as a disease that affected not just one part of my body but my entire physical and psychological well-being.

I noticed that the lymph nodes under my right arm would suddenly flare up and become painful. This was always triggered by a pain in my throat. I asked the oncologist whether there were any drugs to boost my immune system; he suggested that I might like to try homoeopathy. After reading a couple of books on the subject I made an appointment at the Royal Homoeopathic Hospital in London. Six years before I would have dismissed homoeopathy as quackery but now I had decided to overcome my scepticism and keep an open mind.

'We don't claim to be able to cure cancer,' the doctor at the hospital explained, 'but research has shown an improvement in survival rates when a drug called iscador is used as complementary therapy with conventional treatments.' 'Iscador is derived from mistletoe and is a poison that works by stimulating the body's natural defences. It's also possible that it helps to kill some cancerous cells.' I decided to try it and went back to the hospital every day for a week to learn how to give myself iscador injections, which had to be administered three times a week. The doctor also recommended aromatherapy for relaxation, so every six weeks I would see the aromatherapist for an hour of massage using different oils. The sessions helped me to control the pain in my arm and shoulder and left me feeling pleasantly relaxed. At home, I often used the lavender oil she recommended in my bath.

Two weeks after Easter I started my journalism course. At first it was exhausting, but doing it gave me a sense of achievement and purpose and my days once more had a structure. While I had been at home before the operation and recovering afterwards I had felt cut off and isolated. My life had seemed aimless and all the days the same: I would spend the morning cleaning the flat, take a walk down the shops to buy a newspaper, and then sleep for most of the afternoon. I envied my friends who were working and longed to live normally again. Now I felt less lethargic and more energetic. My appetite had improved and I was gaining weight.

When I asked the surgeon if the cancer would come back following the removal of my lymph nodes he said, 'It's like standing under a dark cloud. It may rain, but there again, the cloud may just blow away.' Of course, he did not know the answer to my question. I do not know either. Cancer is unpredictable and I would never be so arrogant as to claim that I have beaten it completely. It has become my stalker. I watch out for it over my shoulder. We try to hide from each other. At the moment, it is a stalemate.

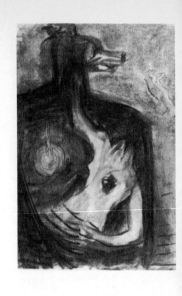

Anubis

Riverroad, Meandering Root

Hilda Raz

REPAIR

In my house, men tear out the floor:
hammering, then wood splits –
hour on hour. You almost need
safety glasses for this work, the blond says
and truly, as I go for the phone,
the kitchen is now rubble. Delight
a paste bubble in my throat. If anger is tangible
here it is, a danger to these men
who let fly plaster, the smell of something old
letting go. They unmake what I made
with my life, or where I made it.

LET'S CONSIDER THE CONSEQUENCES

only,
the damage,
the number of bricks cracked
in the passageway, doors swollen
by water-rot, frames to pare down,
mildew to scour, how much
to seal up, or seal out.
                    Let's count, yes, quantify
so we can sort the pile of damp clothing, the
discarded underwear with stains, the breakfast napkins
to hang out, hang on line the number of bodily fluids, mixed,
the shrinking lengths of divisions, weights of bias ...

Now you have a notebook, pages filled with digits, the sweet
wise voice of the wire turning, connecting, recommending
    measure, a count,
the quantifying of the salt and the sugar,
                         'Well, now
you have the damage report, the bottom line, the sum.
Consider the lilies of the field, how they sway in wind
without reference to your pages, how little they care
for laughter or the dour voice, the smile tucked under the chin,
the complaint, the whine, how – if nothing else – you have
your dear cornea, lungs that puff and inflate their wings, lucky
muscle of the calf, the knee, if we could cut an oval and put
the celluloid disc in place how we would see movement, the
    universe
shifting and settling down in its elliptical orbit, add the catch
    in the stars
the breath makes.'

So you are advised to burn the notebook, its pages,
the maps and wire measure of damage and move on, move
    along
until what happens is only a measure of forgetting, detaching
distress, your upset, your dyspepsia from the air of the
    orchard.
Move ahead and not refer, never refer to
anything other than the sweet taste in your mouth of breath,
the steady blood beat, the road hot and loud under your feet,
    infinite.

WEATHERING/BOUNDARIES/WHAT IS GOOD

Your silence, your hands, skin, your mouth.
On the telephone, sleepy, the son of my body.
The sun on my body. His alarm clock ringing. His birthday.
She, matter-of-fact, cool, saying what she knows, promising
to discover what she doesn't at the library. Daughter
of my body, Persephone and I Demeter. You with your $125
worth of spring bulbs divided three ways, three friends, three
graces. We plant them together,
warm earth in the garden where your mother watches,
who has cancer too. I make stew –
you bring veggies I cook with meat – and rice custard. You
    build
onto our patio garden. The patio is rich and crunchy with
    acorns.
Cat and I stand on the driveway – warm – to find Orion. Now
you are naked and sleeping as I write. Dear God, keep us safe.
My breast is healing well.
I am supple of body. My spirit what? Still at home in my body.

Cancer is one of the few internal diseases that can be cured.
I am a person who has cancer now.

You show me fronds of prairie grasses, beige\lavender in sun
in your garden – sun, sun all day – in high 70s – on your
   garden.
On ours.

Waiting for oncologist with you, v. scared. I'm still me, same me
no matter what he says. Biopsy report shocks me. You say, 'So
you know more than the doctor?' – you with me all afternoon,
read report with me. Necrotic tissue. Adjacent cells abnormal.
We go shopping, for a walk. His nurse says, 'Recovery is
partially dependent …' on my attitude. I buy an expensive purse
in the shape of a pouch, what's missing in my body, that last
year's thievery. She speaks about her dream of ribbons and
banners, floating upward into light,
and her ecstatic sense of losing individual boundaries, losing
them and merging them into the natural universe. I am fascinated
and afraid.

M U

'… the old root giving rise to mystery was *mu*, with cognates
MYSTICAL and MUTE. MYSTERY came from the Greek
muein with the meaning of closing the lips, closing the eyes.'
Lewis Thomas

Misery a block in the head
a block I hum mmmm through, the way *mother*
mmmm helps me move to. Umber attaches to shadows
in hedge-ribbons. Feet mmmmmmmm, hit-sounds like murder
stitched to lips, the miles, humm, eyes shut shuttered, cement
walk studded with dark I'm afraid mmmmmo
and now I am come alone at midnight onto the pineneedles of
   the park.

I am come to say goodbye in the dark but my mouth won't open.
What opens is my eye to the open edge of the metal tunnel under
the curve of the spiral slide I'm afraid to rise to. I'm standing at
the base to cry out at midnight Whose children will come down?
Who bashes into my arms so we open our mouths to this
cadence no no no no mmm mommy up again to ride the big slide
she and I falling into the dark air. Open is the mouth of the metal
tunnel.
Tomorrow, mmmmu, the knife.

BREAST/FEVER

My new breast is two months old,
gel used in bicycle saddles
for riders on long-distance runs,
stays cold under my skin
when the old breast is warm;
catalogue price, $276. My serial number,
#B-1754, means some sisters under the skin.
My new breast
my new breast is sterile,
will never have cancer.

Once every sixty years
according to the Chinese calendar
comes the year of the golden horse.
Over me your skin is warm,
sweetgel, ribbontongue, goldhorse.
You suck the blank to goosebumps.

HowmIgonnaget there when you're gone
back to your youngthing, sweetcurl?
He moans over your back
twitching your buttons raw. My scar

means nothing to him, a mapletwirl
a whirligig, your center and maypole.

Death waits in the book, the woods,
the TV, the helicopter blades merging
over the house, your hair a fine curl
mist over your haunches, smooth hook near.
You'll curl red over him when I'm under
the ash, gone, all mind or nothing.
Who the hell loves a tree?

Don't tell me on the phone your voice
a fine ringing replica of mine that you've
got sickies, fever, ticks from the job
you won't worry about don't I either
you nut, you bitch dog mother I bred you
out of leaves and mash my blood on the floor
my liver colored placenta curled in a cold bowl.
Who do you think you are with my sick breasts
on your chest. Oh God let me live to touch her
working out the next generation of women.

PETTING THE SCAR
for Alicia Ostriker

You know what? I don't want a brave death,
faithful children mopping up after my body,
sweet thing, nubbly fissures and skin so soft
it's silklike. Let my daughter wail at the side
of her lover's bed, her heart in its tough covering
beating powdery as a butterfly's wing.
My son, oh no, let him turn up his torso
to the Greek sun, his heartscar sexy, raised
on his dark skin.

So what are we to do tonight, finished with passion,
roaming our rooms, our thumbs hooked
under the spines of books, notebooks by each chair,
forbidden smokes flushed and fats scoured away?
You tell me to reach under my shirt and pet the scar.

Did you hear about the lozenge of blood on the binding
of our friend's new book, who is trying hard in a far country?
I forgot to tell you. 'If I can bear to touch it,' she said.
'Yet,' surely you'd add.

Under my robe – I must put down my pen to do it –
my palm finds chill: this is not a metaphor
but an image, true, a fact: I swear it.
No pouty lip the color of eyelids. A cold blank.

But the scar!
Riverroad, meandering root, stretched coil, wire chord, embroidery
in its hoop, mine, my body.

Oh, love!

FISH-BELLY-MOUND

Press in hard to hurt
nine times, twice or more
with your thumb,
the other hand on
that puffed up place.
Thumb rigid and forefinger
a rictus. Tight fist,
fingers merged. Now

peace will flood you,
an overwash from some
ocean of light.

We lay head to toe, neighbors
on tables for treatment, both ill,
both having lost too much to mention.

The side of my body, numb forever,
my clothes hid, still drifted on.
He smiled through a red beard
as our attendants strapped on electrodes.
And the while his naked foot jerked
and kicked and we talked, I pressed
and pressed and now have come home
to shadows where I flail and sink
in light these words swim through,
my fingers a net he tried to weave.

FOR BARBARA, WHO BRINGS A GREEN STONE IN THE SHAPE OF A TRIANGLE

From ocean
this porous shape
indisputably green
color I tell you
of healing, the color
I have chosen around me
like a vapor, this towel
on my shoulders, its green
drape an air over my scar,
then a shirt I pull over my head
and let fall for the green
lint-shed filaments of healing, moss

some ancestor might bind up with spit
and press onto my breast, no, the space
where my breast has been.
                     Yesterday
for the space of an hour, a woman
came here with her child, raised
up shirt, her breast was flesh.
The child pulled where her nipple
is, and touched his mouth
to her and filled himself.
She talked as he drank.
I listened to nipple,
a hiss of milk.
Miracle.

In your photos of green ocean
and boats, a line of women in green air,
their arms muscular, pulls against green water.
Their breasts are bare.
One, yours, shows a faint scar
my skin wears.
                In the past year
I have given up four of the five organs
the body holds to call itself woman.
                       Green
healer, today my body carries
in its clever hand the triangle
sea gave up to you
and you gave me.
                   I press it to my chest,
empty of nipple, of milk, of nurture,
and feel you there: friend, lover
of women, teacher. You speak to me
each green vowel of the life language.

MAPPING/BLEATING

I think chemistry has much to gain from reviving the personal, the emotional, the stylistic core of the struggle to discover and create the molecular world.
  – *Roald Hoffman, 'Under the Surface of the Chemical Article'*

The graphic depiction of molecules … Hoffmann argues, is so central to the science of chemistry that its conventions and ambiguities deserve reflection. A chemist faces the same difficulty as a landscape painter: how to represent three-dimensional shapes in two dimensions.

  – *Emily Grosholz, 'Roald Hoffmann's Praise of Synthetic Beauty'*

My fingers, mine, *my* fingers
instructed as ice molecules
in trees, now on this airplane wing out the window,
to address the subject of
no, not war (planes and missiles
we pop as objects on the nightly news,
the morning news we set our short wave
scanner to)
but death, a subject
breathing
used to seem to catch up to
and expand as atoms of air, pure ether.

My fingers move at random, push
the words out on this paper. Fog
smothers the wing tip. I can't see lights.
Am dizzy.

Where are we going? You are moving radon
gas over the sensor box. He buckles the web.
She tucks the head of a newborn (thumbs
a half moon around each apricot ear) under her rib. I am
aloft, yes, tucked in. I am going to smell,
no, say right, apprehend death, its
molecules in cells cut out,
excised; only a prim removal
of some feeder flesh, her breast. Mine's
gone so I'm immune. My friend gives me this gift
of witness. Once there, I'll hold her daughter's ear. Going,
my chest is laved in apricot lotion under the linen of my shift.

What next? A band of clay braided at the lip
of the gift cup wrapped in my underwear,
milk spotted with chocolate floaters, or brandy in steam, tea
    steeped until mash of pattern
predicts the final outcome: death. When we land on earth
first thing is, I'll unpack this stoneware cup, brew comfort.
Still, to be honest, down small or up here,
the light plaids, curtains golden on cotton, and I'm bleating.

BERNINI'S RIBBON
– an aerial sculpture by S. Roth-Kent

Someone else's voice in this lobby,
clear but unfamiliar, 'I was an executive secretary
before I went to med school,'
and again a familiar male voice saying,
'You don't *get* it, do you?' – the female tag
at the end of the sentence, 'do you?' –
as in *The Exorcist* when a small girl opens
her mouth and out comes the voice
of the devil like musk, a shock.

175

Getting personal with someone new,
unfamily, unknown, someone to help, to help
you.
      So in the course of the day's spiral
from garble comes story: she was healing
at last, the edges of the crust dissolving in warm
water, surface only one foreground of many
textures, only one shiny surface leading the eye
out and away until color takes over the job,
lifts with purples and golds and sulfur, galls
the eye up to the proscenium arch, the ceiling
higher beyond, and Bernini's Ribbon
through high air a dropped clue
to follow: voices, the maze.

NUTS

to success. The third day lucky
on the job and nothing's changed: I work all day,
I worked all day. Nuts to beauty.
Bikini, music, then the childbed. Inside out
through the door of a birdcage: Margaret Atwood.
Now in the mirror, a sea turtle with goiter.

Nuts to the mirror.
Forty below windchill, she rides her bike
to work, is hit by a truck. Who's freezing
on the radiator is bound to freeze.
Nuts to visitors. They slip on ice like thunder,
clap closed their wimples, rise, then sue.

What's nibbling your liver, kid?
Birdsong. Nuts to praise,
the poet's contract, nuts to quicksilver

in glass, nuts to the fever it measures,
the belly's gripe, nuts to love that only
smells like a vine, to bougainvillea on the tongue,
to ice cream, to blood warm on the palm, nuts
to surgery, the pain it stops, the pain it is.

WHO DOES SHE THINK SHE IS

Risen from the cart,
the sick bed, the steel trolley?
Witch of the world, her roars
hide in waterfalls so small
no human on earth has seen them.

Small, I wander the paths
of the world, dust, a miracle
nose to scoop air, breathing.
Between my skin and spine a thin layer
of cells, a silence.

Who do I think I am,
a solitude, a poor bridge, small beer?
Enough that my eyes focus
on that emerald tree, that spruce,
blue in its huge dying.

Risen again, once more
the heat of my skin
pours radiance, praise,
salt and hops into air, my skin a bracelet
of psalms, my navel invisible, a veil.

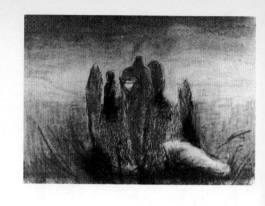

Standing Stones

Many Voices

Debbie Dickinson

Movement – the rhythm. Cancer exists for a reason – not just one, but many reasons – it offers a clue to our life journey. It's the voice that needs to be listened to, and when we stop and listen we may hear not one, but many voices. Not all as loud as each other, not all at the same time, but layered – the layers of who we are.

This book has taken over five years to put together. Contributors have died along the way; friends have died too. My own contribution spans this period of time. Months go by when I never look at, or even think about the book, but each time I come back to it, more experiences, more thoughts, more voices and more ideas inform my writing. I realise that this piece is not only an account of my cancer experience, but that through the exercise of finding the right voice and the right rhythm with which to write, I have created a window into the very essence of who I am.

Initially, I tried to write my story using one voice but this felt hollow and limited. I wrote another account but that felt abstract, cold; too tonal. So I tried to combine the voices, but how could I make harmony when chaos resides? I started to think of myself as music, to feel the loneliness and vulnerability of a solitary instrument, but also to feel the beauty of the lone instrument as it emerges out of the accompaniment, out of the warmth and support that comes through the embrace of the other instruments – when the passage of music is completed and the moment is right.

Through relating to the different emotions and aspects that create who I am as instruments and musical elements – as in jazz – I found a new way of looking at the different voices and layers within myself. From these I began to build a framework within which to share my story. I realised that my whole being could be seen as a musical metaphor.

I believe that my cancer is not a virus, not an invasion from outside, that it is not linked to an environmental cause. I see it rather as cells 'out of sync' with each other – the cancer cells reproducing faster than other cells, out of step with other cell growth – rogue cells in the community of cells that make up my body. I believe that cancer is illogical and unpredictable and in direct conflict with order and structure. I cannot impose order on what is essentially a chaotic experience. The choices I have in dealing with it are as infinite as my life choices.

I challenge the cause-and-effect approach to illness, which by its very nature embraces a linear perspective of time. I will not make myself write this story from the beginning and create an ending because that is the 'logical' consequence of a beginning. And I will not see the cancer as an 'effect' and thereby create a 'cause'. Nor do I accept that it is my 'fault', or, the opposite, that I am a victim and it just 'happened to me', as a result of past experiences or bad luck or whatever else. I do believe that I shape my own personal reality and I do want to 'own' my cancer experience.

My belief is not that I am 'Debbie with cancer', but that I am Debbie with many healthy cells, and I attempt to focus on and direct strength towards those healthy cells. I try to balance a belief that often occupies a difficult place between denial, and acknowledgement of the importance and seriousness of cancer; not overly focusing on the cancer itself but looking at the cancer as existing within my healthy body.

So now I offer you my story in different voices, with their own rhythm, and leave you to hear what you will.

The story can unfold as a drama; a series of events. Events which happened to me, events for which I am responsible. It is also a story of hope and of despair. It is a story of defeat and of conquest, of denial and of self discovery, of selflessness and self-indulgence. It is a story of calm and of panic – it is all these things all of the time.

Here in 1993, I have had cancer for five years and I still find it incredibly difficult to write about, to have an overview of an ongoing experience. When I am immersed in the experience, I write in my journal. These writings become a part of the experience, a sharing of fragments of thoughts and insights with a potential reader. When I am outside the experience the last thing I want to do is think about it because the cancer is so integrated, so much a part of me, assimilated into the core of my being. When I read back my writings they often feel to me a little detached and cold.

Sometimes, through an event, I realise how much I've changed and I feel amazed. Recently I had a birthday party – a small gathering of very close and dear friends. It was the first time for years that I had positively wanted to surround myself with close friends – just for me. Towards the end of a wonderful barbecue we sat around talking, and a couple of very old friends started reminiscing about my wildness, my flamboyance and happy-go-lucky attitude to life. I was amazed that this was me they were talking about – I realised that I felt very removed from that wild young woman, but also that I felt proud of her, and honoured to have known her.

Now, I feel secure enough in who I am to be able to start to let her talk and be again. To let her coexist with the maturity and experience that I now have and not feel scared that she will make me fall into 'bad habits' again: avoidance tactics, excess consumption of drugs, booze and so on. I felt elated by the gathering and by my own personal history and excited by being 36, with all that experience to draw on.

I realise now that I am coming out of a tunnel, or reaching a plateau, or whatever image is appropriate to the incredible self-growth that has happened within me over the last few years. Sometimes I feel so removed from the cancer that I think I must have imagined it, and the whole five-year experience seems like a dream. At other times it is so real that everything else is overshadowed by it, as it looms like a tree in full bloom.

Why? The question so familiar to cancer patients and their loved ones – 'Extremely unusual in someone so young...' '– The bladder of a 75-year-old man in a 30-year-old woman ...' – even the medics ask why.

Given no rational explanation, I believed that it must be MY fault. It must be my lifestyle, my blocked emotions – I was never very good at expressing my feelings. And then there's my diet – very erratic – and of course, years of sex and drugs and rock 'n' roll – God punishes those who have a good time. And then there's my personality – a definite cancer type. Oh, and don't forget my unresolved childhood issues and my current lifestyle and too much work – workaholism, even. And there's probably also a dose of moral retribution lurking in the background, due to my perceived 'sexual deviancy' as a lesbian.

So of course I should eat brown rice, and go straight to therapy for my personality and childhood issues, and get rid of the stress by reducing my workload. But wait a minute – this solution seems to imply that it's all a case of cause and effect – yet isn't this supposed to be the holistic, alternative attitude towards cancer?

I try to balance this with the orthodox attitude – 'let's go in and zap the cancer growth' – which can ignore the *meaning* of illness, focusing solely on the effect. From this standpoint, it doesn't really matter why we've got it, or even that the doctors don't actually know what they are doing with it. Cancer can't possibly hold useful information – best to just blast the tumours away and see if they grow back. So many conflicting thoughts and ideas. Sometimes, I haven't known what, or even how to think.

Very early in my experience, I remember being visited by a 'friend of a friend', a woman who had miraculously managed to recover from cancer and wanted to share her story with me and inspire me to use her method of healing, which was by painting her life. First she went back to her birth and painted her life forwards, then she painted it back-wards, then forwards again – in a totally linear fashion. This worked for her, but was anathema to me. I do not know how she instinctively arrived at this method, but she healed herself without drastic surgery. Now she runs classes in her approach; she is happy and has found her own way. That is all any of us can hope for. But my way is not linear. For me there are no beginnings and endings – just infinity.

A few years after this meeting, a very close friend was diagnosed as having cancer. We had always been like two sides of a coin in our atti-tudes to life. Although we often chose different routes and ideas, we respected and understood each other's viewpoints. Her approach to her life with cancer was very different from mine. Where I drew comfort from psychics she rejected their ideas. Where I was wary of orthodox approaches she embraced them. One day, a few months before she died, we talked about death and I realised that I was essentially influenced by my belief that there is some kind of afterlife. My friend believed that once we died the 'lights were turned off', and this belief gave her a fierce desire to hold on to her life as she knew it, and to continue her life work making excellent television documentaries.

As we talked, I realised that neither of us was right or wrong. For her, maybe death was the end of her existence and maybe it was not the end for me. I suddenly realised how personal our journeys really are, and that there are no rules. Although I am still here to tell my story and she is not, I feel no satisfaction. I feel as if our arguments are unresolved.

However, one night shortly after her death, I was driving alone and thinking deeply of her. It was a winter night, with the kind of mist evocative of a Sherlock Holmes film. In my head I was going over our conversations and I said to myself or out loud: 'So Shauna, I can't even ask you to tell me if you were right. Because if you were, then you've gone and if you weren't, you're probably too busy being surprised to come and tell me.' Suddenly, as if the lights had been turned on around me, my head was full of brightness and I felt an incredible silence and calm. My mind's eye was filled with what I can only describe as a lake, so still – absolutely no movement or sound – a nothingness filled with total peace and quiet – totally complete in itself. This lasted for a couple of minutes and then I became aware of the hustle and bustle around me and inside me as the sensation lifted. But I was left with the incredible realisation that perhaps there is an end to eternity, and that when the time is right and we have had as many lives as is our destiny, then maybe the lights as we know them do go out. I don't know anything for sure, except that at that moment the Universe showed me that there is peace – and that nothing is indeed something.

I believe that cancer comes into our lives undirected. We can choose how to perceive it and our perception changes, as if organically, through the passage of time. No one knows for certain why it comes, why it goes, what it is. At this moment in time, 16 June 1993, I am convinced that my 'unexplainable' cancer is rooted in the non-physical sphere – that my cancer is not primarily a physical force, but is a symptom of a soul malady.

And sometimes the safest place for me is in the cancer itself. Sometimes, I feel like it is my secret lover, my bottle of gin, my comforter, my way out. When I think of it as an addiction, I get a completely different perspective on my relationship to it. Then I'm scared of the power with which I am drawn to the danger of living with this loaded pistol so close. Russian Roulette seems tame in comparison.

The stress involved in living with cancer is enormous.

Cancer as an addiction – what a thought. Yet – it offers me the comfort of the secret affair, the means to escape, an excuse for only dealing with what is real and immediate in life, fantasies surrounding different death scenes, a removal from the mundane matters of life, a release from the physical sphere on to an elevated plane – all factors are at play in my experience with cancer.

And I have known the process of letting go of the focus of the addiction during the period of recovery. I have realised that no one can cure me, no one can heal me, no one can do it for me. Only I can do it. – Aren't these the necessary realisations for a recovering addict?

I could go to groups or read books but the patterns and dependencies would remain. I believe now that if I had the cancer cut out and continued with my life as normal, putting the experience behind me, filing it away as a memory and not entering the spiritual sphere of the experience, I would be denying myself in some way. But when faced with life or death choices, holding on to this spiritual sphere can become harder.

I believe that if I was an alcoholic and gave up drink through control and willpower alone, I would not have achieved a true spiritual recovery. Yet other people stop drinking and put it behind them, and have successful operations or treatments and put these behind them too; possibly that is all they need to take from their experience. I suspect that if in the first two years of my cancer I had gone to the hospital and had the tumours removed and was clear of the illness, I would probably have taken that option too. Consequently I would have had another set of experiences and a different life. Sometimes I wonder how it would feel to be able to put all one's faith in the medical system, or in a miracle cure, or in one's own willpower – but deep in myself I know this is not an option for me.

I feel I must explore the reasons why I continue to grow these tumours, while trying not to punish myself for them. I have a need to understand although I now think that when I can truly accept the excitement of self-discovery, of meeting fears head on, for its own sake – when this replaces my need to find a cause, a reason, a justification for pursuing my journey of self-discovery – then I will be able to let go of any remnants of the addiction and just accept my different voices and layers and allow them to coexist.

My cancer experience is an ongoing process. I not only think of the cancer as significant for what has been, but also for what is to come.

Maybe now it is more significant for my future, in helping me to prepare for what will happen in my future life.

Cancer is not always central in my life now. Some days go by and I don't think about it at all, but then I remember and I feel anxious. When immersed in the 'cancer experience', directly engaged with it either through treatment or general lifestyle, I'm so busy dealing with it that I don't have the time to be stressed.

However, in December 1992 I felt incredible stress at the prospect of the next hospital visit. I had been clear of tumours on the previous two visits. But I didn't know if I really was clear or if this was a pause, a honeymoon period. I needed to be clear for five years to feel confident; this was now one year.

These phases are hard; waiting, not knowing, forgetting, then remembering. As the hospital visits get closer I feel ill, exhausted, I have migraine, leg aches. I have to learn to live with the stress, the loss of libido, the not knowing, the feeling of potential claustrophobia caused by this small time bomb. And I can't run from this. It's not like being able to change jobs, or move house, or end a relationship because I feel trapped. This is an internal trap and I'm making it all by myself. This is a powerful lesson for a claustrophobic. I have to take the cancer with me everywhere: it's inside, constant. I face the challenge of transforming my stress into something else – of learning to change while staying in one place. I need to explore my claustrophobia, my fears of being trapped, and to expose the patterns in my life that have developed as a result of these fears.

I have also identified the fact that my drive and adventurousness towards life are fuelled not solely by a curiosity about what is around the next corner, but also by the sense of a hand pushing me from behind. With the acknowledgement of this fear of being stopped and becoming trapped has come the realisation that I have a deep ambivalence to life itself.

How comforting it is to believe that I might die at the age of 40, as my mother did. Opting out of longevity means that I avoid dealing with any of the issues that confront women as they get older. I remember a couple of years ago visiting a psychic healer and asking her if I would die young of cancer. She laughed, and said 'No way. There's not going to be an easy exit for you – you're here for the ride.' Now I understand what she meant. Now I'm letting go of the idea of dying young. I'm here to stay.

I contemplate the fact that I'm 35 and my body is filling out, my reproductive years are drawing to a close. I don't like the way my body is changing; the fullness of my women's hips, the rounding thighs, the loose upper arms. My face is lined: lived in on a good day, creased on a bad day. Ageing is a reality. And I am going to live and to grow old.

Now I've told you some of my evolving attitudes, dreams and thoughts. Maybe it would be useful to go back to when it first started – to remember what happened in 1988, eight years ago:

I had worked in the music business as a general fixer and doer, sound engineer and tour manager, for a number of years. Before I became ill, I'd lived and breathed a particular music project inspired by an ideal-istic dream of women visibly defying their own limitations and the world's expectations. I was part of an all-women jazz group in the mid-1980s and we shared the same dreams. We toured the world and fought for our right to be seen and to be taken seriously, both as women and jazz musicians.

As manager and sound engineer, I set up the tours and organized all the gigs. I was a woman with a mission. People responded to our energy and to the beliefs and ideals that we held. We achieved things others said were impossible, breaking endless new ground, and sharing an intense, varied and exhausting five years together. The group gave me the opportunity to give myself entirely to something. It provided me with the family I'd never had, it tested my limits, challenged me and gave purpose to my life. I could travel the world with a reason; it gave me a sense of identity. My whole life was tied up with the group and I shared the experience with a most loving, important friend and lover for those five years.

I put the group and my work first and I ignored my own creative needs. I didn't know how to take time off for myself or how to replenish my energies, how to relax, how to take care of my soul. I felt frustrated, but I was waiting for my lover to make a decision for me, to change our lifestyle. Then I started to feel ill and incredibly tired and gradually my declining health meant the decision was taken out of our hands.

One of the earliest and most significant experiences I underwent as a result of the cancer was realising the difference between 'self' and 'identity'. Quite soon after being diagnosed, I was lying in a hospital bed when I came to the harsh and frightening realisation that I defined exactly who I was in the world by what I did. Now that I was no longer able to work in the same way, my sense of who I was became incredibly shaky. The essence of who I am, that part of me that connects to my soul – my 'self' – had been neglected in favour of the part that worked in the world – my 'identity'. My well-defined sense of identity did not equal a well-defined sense of self.

Being ill had stripped me of the active, ego-defined being I and my peers knew so well, and left me with a rather more naked and unsophisticated 'self'. It was especially hard to cope with the difficulty of loved ones in dealing with the change in me – from coping, positive Debbie to the insecure, rather fearful being that I now was from time to time. Now I realise that I can only give myself in a healthy way to something if I am centred and balanced in myself. In the past I was not, and the outcome was detrimental to my health and general well-being. I became ill whilst experiencing an overwhelming sense of feeling lost and an inability to direct my own life.

At first I suffered from physical debilitation and perpetual exhaustion. I was 30 years old, yet I felt finished – worn out. I had constant migraines, hangovers, aches and pains. Was I to believe my acupuncturist when she said that I couldn't treat my body as if I was a 20-year-old? I know I lived fast, but this was ridiculous.

Then I began peeing blood. I was lucky to have a GP who recommended all the hospital tests, determined to find out what was wrong.

The final test was a cysoctomy. When the consultant looked inside my bladder he exclaimed that it looked more like the bladder of a 75-year-old man than a 30-year-old woman.

Fortunately I ended up with a medic who enthuses about his area of work and invents new means of doing investigative surgery. When he operates he gives his patients a cocktail of drugs rather than the general anaesthetic favoured by other consultants. I was able to look into my bladder through an eyeglass, and I saw an extraordinary floating plant, like a seaweed, attached to the side of the bladder, floating comfortably and occupying a third of the space. No wonder I'd been toxic – I had blocked drains!

The medic took this growth away by inserting a telescope inside a wire through the urethra and into the bladder. The thin wire held an electrical current and they literally 'zapped' the tumours, burning them off with electricity. As I understand it, this results in the burnt area then growing back as scar tissue, on which the rumours tend not to grow. However the doctors have no idea, and from what I've gathered no interest, in what long-term effects this scar tissue could have on the overall functioning of the bladder lining.

After this first operation I was told to come back in three months so the consultant could have another look and see if any new tumours had grown. At this stage we did not know how serious things were. I went back for the results of the tests a few weeks later and discovered that I had a malignant tumour. However, there was still a chance that it was only an isolated growth. No such luck – over the next year I went back at three-monthly intervals, and each time more tumours had grown. These would be burnt off, and then grow back, always in a different place. Nobody knew why – it was extremely unusual in one so young.

Then came the day when the doctor told me that I had now developed bladder cancer rather than individual tumours, and that the speed of the growth was surprisingly aggressive. Now, the whole bladder lining was volatile, showing masses of potential tumours. I suppose the change was similar to going from having a few pimples to having acne, but with rather more serious consequences.

Although other medics would have suggested a more drastic approach, such as surgery, fortunately for me my consultant recommended I continue with the three-monthly cysotomies and the removal of the tumours, combined with a course of localized chemotherapy. He explained how fortunate I was in not having to have a general anaesthetic every time, and told me not to worry as he had known cases where people had had this course of treatment for five years or so – although, of course, most of these were over 60, so if they eventually had surgery it wasn't such a big deal! Not such a big deal for who, I wondered!

That day I had gone to the hospital alone, as I always did – I had always thought it better to deal with these things alone. Need equalled weakness in my book. Dependency was unacceptable. I was streetwise and tough. I sat there quietly, barely hearing what he was saying – 'aggressive', 'cancer', 'chemo', 'surgery' – it all sounded like a bad dream. When he had finished I said 'thank you' and left. I got back to my car and just sat there and shook all over. Suddenly I felt terror. I realised that I'd been in denial for a year or more, in 'carry on anyway' mode.

I had been taking Chinese herbs. I had been having regular acupuncture. I had cleaned up my diet, I'd stopped smoking. But despite these changes I had not really registered what having cancer actually meant to me. Suddenly, the vulnerability of my bladder – and indeed my whole life – struck me. The ease with which I could lose my bladder, indeed even die; the fear of getting caught up in a cycle of medical treatment, side effects, hospitals, doctors; the loss of my physical independence, the quality of existence as I knew it – all suddenly hit me. Why was I growing these tumours? No one knew and the reasons didn't seem to be of any great interest or importance to the medics.

I was scared, and at this stage unaware that I could choose, that orthodox medicine was only an option; no more sophisticated or 'right' than any other approach to illness. Although I had been pursuing alternative therapies, orthodox medicine still had the superior status in my mind.

So to the next stage: the invasive treatment – the chemo. Coming off the street every week for three months, walking into the ward, having a tube inserted through my urethra into my bladder, hoping that I wouldn't get an inexperienced or nervous nurse who couldn't do it properly. Then the discomfort of lying there for two hours, feeling like I was going to burst as I held the liquid in; the bruising; the burning; and then up again and home. Feeling violated, deadening off half my body to deal with the invasion. The effects of that on my sexual being. The psychic assault. I didn't believe that there was any way that part of my body could be poisoned without me feeling it in the rest of my being.

The chemo had a profound emotional effect on me. I realise now that up to this point I had seen the tumours as something dirty, something growing beyond my control. I didn't think of the cancer as coming from outside, or as an outside poison or illness. I could see that the tumours were part of me – that I was making them. The revulsion I felt for them was a revulsion towards my own body, particularly from the waist down. The chemo accentuated those feelings. I had to block the feeling of my body being invaded and violated by the treatment, in order to welcome the poisoning of that one part of my body – I thought that I had to believe that my bladder was an enemy in some way.

I tried to be positive by meditating on positive images such as envisaging the liquid as light and the process as cleansing. But that wasn't what was happening. The reality was that I felt the chemo was a violent poison and could only work by declaring war on my cells – all my cells. The Chinese say 'fight a big force with another big force'; the doctors say 'go in and obliterate the enemy'. But neither of them say what happens to your psyche when you declare war on part of yourself.

I came to realise that a distinct quality of my cancer is that the cancer cells are a creation of my own biorhythms: that my cancer is the result of some cells being out of time, out of step, out of rhythm with the rest of the cells. Once I 'owned' the cancer as part of me, and took on board all that that means, things started to change. I started to own the feelings I had for my body, and to realise how much I felt encumbered by my body. Up to that point my head had ruled; my body was an unwanted necessity to pull around, to abuse from time to time. I would see it as an obstacle, sometimes standing in the way of my achievement with its pathetic limitations and need for rest. Gradually I realised just how much my life had been determined by my need to test my own limits.

Up to this point, I had lived my life intuitively. I had always dreamed and hoped and believed that I could do anything if I really wanted to – what was important was the dream or vision, not my limitations. The flavour of a dream would penetrate my life and act as a subconscious directive, and at key moments I would have the strong feeling that 'this is right – this is where I should be'.

The worst part of this stage of the cancer was the loss of this ability to dream. Whenever I started to dream an ironclad hand would come down, as if holding down my spirit. It was awful. My life felt colourless and hopeless. It seemed the only 'relevant' dream I could have was of being tumour-free. But this felt like basing a dream on winning a game of Russian Roulette – it felt too out of control. I found it really hard to believe that I could shape my own reality while losing confidence in my body, not feeling that I could rely on my health anymore. I hadn't truly realised that health *is* the most precious gift that we have, and that the body we occupy is a gift, and a means through which we can experience enormous pleasure.

My mother died at 40, when I was eight years old. Throughout the years I knew her she had been unhappy and ill, and an alcoholic. I had inherited a very negative view of her, and felt deep within myself the total absence of a mother. Through having cancer, I have been able to experience different feelings about her; a deep hurt and longing and a strong identification with her self-destructive tendencies. I feel it is a tragedy that I wasn't taught the value of her memory. The memory of her that had been handed to me was of somebody best forgotten; an unfortunate phase of my father's life. This was, in effect, a total negation of an essential aspect of my life story. How can I love myself, feel good about myself, if I am ambivalent about the very source that gave me life? How can I feel good about myself as a whole being when I cut off or hate one part of my body?

Now I feel the tragedy of her life, the helplessness and frustration she must have felt from years of pain, both self-induced and through illness; her loneliness, her disillusionment, her isolation, despair and self-defeat. What were her dreams? Did she want to be a singer? a poet? a dreamer? Why did she give up on her life? I realise that not only do I have the wounds of my own inner child to heal, my own child's voice to listen to, I have my mother's too.

When I was about 14, I realised that I could either become bitter and twisted about my childhood or I could love and forgive. I chose the latter. But in rising above the pain to embrace understanding and rationalization, I left the little girl behind. I also forgot – or never knew – that part of being mothered is about receiving tenderness. In the absence of my mother, I also had the absence of tenderness. As an adult I have experienced similar feelings of abandonment – normally when love affairs have ended. Sometimes I feel as if I carry around a bin full of feelings of abandonment and when a few more come along the bin must shed some of the bottom layers to make room for the new ones. Certainly my life had lurched from emotional crisis to emotional crisis. But I have learnt through love relationships that I can change this pattern, that I can express feelings without the world coming to an end. Maybe I will even reach the point where I will no longer need the crisis energy of cancer in my life at all.

After the chemo the tumours came back and it looked very likely that surgery was the next option. I made a deal with my medic that I would have no treatment for six months and I would try to heal myself. He agreed, and I stopped everything: acupuncture, herbs, everything. I found a body-orientated therapist and decided to look deep into myself to see why I was growing these tumours. I went on holiday and immersed myself in a beautiful external environment – a sunny tropical paradise in the form of a small island in Thailand. I allowed myself the freedom to examine and question my deep ambivalence about life.

I realised how confused I had become by all the different 'shoulds' and 'shouldn'ts' in connection with cancer and was feeling overwhelmed by the weight of all the possibilities. I didn't know what to attach my belief to; everything seemed to contradict everything else. I thought perhaps I could mix up my own cocktail with a few different approaches, a combination of orthodox and holistic, a complementary approach. But somehow combinations are not the stuff of faith. So I turned to myself. I remained open to the views of others, but started looking to myself to find the key to my own healing. I felt as if I was at a crossroads – one direction would lead deeper into the cancer and the other would lead me deeper into my own journey of self-discovery. I confronted my fears and started the journey and the next time I went to the hospital there were no tumours.

During the year after that hospital visit the tumours came back, but more isolated and consistently less aggressive. Then I had 18 months of no tumours and it seemed as if maybe they really had gone. Although relieved and pleased, I also felt incredibly vulnerable and scared and completely alone. My previously inflated confidence had been punctured like an air cushion. I felt that my mentor, the reason for my journey, my companion, my supporter had gone. The justification I had had for focusing on myself, and not being overwhelmed by the guilt and feelings of selfishness contained in that, had been compromised. Even though I felt that I didn't want or need the cancer, to live without it was scary. I'd got used to it – it was familiar.

Rather than wanting to celebrate, I had an overwhelming need to mourn its passing and to symbolise the change I had undergone through a *rite de passage*, as if freeing a precious bird, or burying a treasure, or letting go of an intimate relationship, or just plain letting go. But I didn't ever feel the right moment.

Then, when I went back to the hospital 12 months later the tumours were back and growing deep into the bladder wall. The operation to remove them was complicated and painful, and the direction of the growth seemed to be changing. For the first time in years, a dangerous question mark hovered over whether or not the cancer was now growing out of my bladder rather than being contained within it.

I was scared that the tumours were so strong, but not surprised at their renewed presence. Somehow I'd known that they hadn't gone. But I had felt that the people who were closest to me had wanted this so much during the previous year that I'd felt uncomfortable mentioning the cancer. I'd felt pushed into saying goodbye before I was ready to, and too guilty about having these feelings to do anything about it. Still, the force with which it re-entered my life shocked me enormously.

I was lucky – the doctors managed to remove the growths before the roots grew into the outside muscle.

AND NOW

Since July 1994, I have made dramatic changes in both my emotional and work relationships. I also go back for a cysoctomy every three to six months. Each time the tumours are there but less firmly rooted, and the doctors are able to remove them and my bladder still works fine.

I feel now that the cancer hovers in both my physical and auric spheres, and I believe that it will stay there until the moment arrives to help it on its eloquent and dignified way, and that this must be done with love and symbolic richness rather than hate and dismissiveness. After all, it is a part of me and just as deserving of memory and gratitude as are all parts of me, and I need to say a respectful goodbye.

This year I hope to go back to my sunny tropical paradise in Thailand and, who knows, maybe I'll say goodbye then.

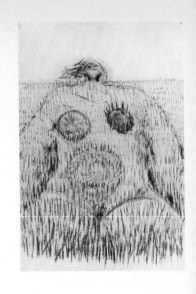

Corn Circles

The Blue Book

Patricia Duncker

I began writing a notebook which I called the Blue Book in a ledger in
November 1975. It was never a journal in the traditional sense. It took
shape from the paper itself: a cash book, a book of accounts, of profit
and loss. The cheapest blank books with hard covers which I could find
at that time were a thick hardboard design, lined paper with a blue
binding. I have gone on writing in these blue books ever since. The Blue
Book is therefore continuous. I wrote down notes, events, landscapes,
poems, bits of poems, reflections, tempers, work plans, ideas, recorded
who I saw, who I met, rebuked myself, other people. Sometimes I wrote
to the people I loved. But nobody ever read the Blue Book. Mostly I
wrote for myself.

Every written life contains gaps, evasions, silences. The Blue Book
was not, and is not, an uncensored space. I have left these gaps there in
the text. But this is not fiction. It is about the world in which we die. Yet
it is part of the unreal world, the world in which we can imagine our
dying. This story concerns one year in my life, which changed me irrevocably. I have not disguised or embroidered upon the events I narrate. I
have learned to mistrust even my own words; for we are not coherent,

consistent beings. But if we are to survive at all we must take responsibility for ourselves, for who we are and for how we decide to act. The Blue Book remains a writing of doubt and ambiguity. It is a place where I tried to understand my own life on my own terms; where I tried to write some fragment of my own raw truth. I am no longer the same woman who wrote this part of the Blue Book. But I remember her; and I acknowledge her as part of myself.

On 11 April 1986 a very tall white man with white hair and a white coat told me that I had cancer. We sat down together and peered at the laboratory report, which was, for me, full of alarming and unintelligible words. The last sentence was the most important and he had underlined it in red ink.

STRONGLY SUGGESTS ARDENOCARCINOMA

I asked him what he proposed to do and whether he could save my life.

I had cancer of the cervix, which might, or might not have spread up the cervical canal into my womb. Cervical cancer, now reaching something like epidemic proportions, particularly among young women, is suspected of being a heterosexually transmitted venereal disease. The structure of the cancer cells suggests a link with warts virus. It is a disease which men pass on to women through penetrative heterosexual intercourse. It is utterly unknown among life-long lesbians and virgin nuns. For half the women who develop the disease it is a fatal consequence of unprotected heterosexual sexual activity. One benefit of the advent of the condom and AIDS education may also be a drop in the incidence of cervical cancer. But for me it was too late.

The very tall white consultant was a surgeon called David Barlow.

'We'll perform a cone biopsy next week,' he said, 'to see how far it's got. And if it's as bad as it looks we'll do a radical hysterectomy followed by radiotherapy and chemotherapy. And that's the treatment.'

'Ah,' I said, giving every appearance of understanding what he said, 'and do you think that you can save my life?'

'You'll be very unlucky if we don't,' he said. Then, seeing that I was firmly contemplating the possibility of being unlucky, he drew upon his war experience for a comparative metaphor.

'It's a bit like the Blitz,' he said, 'you know someone's got to die. But most won't. And you just have to hope it won't be you.'

This element of chance, luck, fate, is always there with any disease. Who survives, who doesn't depends on many things. No doctor dealing with cancer ever makes any promises. Mr Barlow looked at me carefully and then said something which I have always valued ever since.

'It doesn't matter what your attitude is,' he said, 'whether you are very positive or negative about the disease. In my professional experience the attitude of the patient doesn't affect who survives at all.'

For three years before I was told that I had cancer I had been living with my woman lover and a very large tabby cat. It was a stormy triangular relationship. She was a very difficult, petulant, passionate and bad-tempered woman. She was very like the cat, who had preceded her in my affections by some four years. But we were an ambitious household. We were committed to our work, philosophy, writing, teaching, to the small lesbian community among whom we lived, to the politics of radical feminism, to the damp, cold Women's Centre, with its devastating socials and appalling loos, and so, I believed, to each other. While I sat listening to my approaching fate at the hands of the medical profession, she was waiting outside.

Over the following months I experienced much of the treatment meted out to lepers in biblical history. Cancer means death to most women. The Romans placed coins on the eyes of the dead to pay Chaeron's fare across the waters of Lethe on the way to the underworld; and to prevent the dead casting their unseeing eyes upon the living and dragging them, too, away from the kingdom of this world. Some women were afraid to look at me. I embodied their fear. Some women were afraid to touch me; just in case my cancer proved to be contagious.

I made misguided, courageous appearances at the Women's Centre. One young lesbian told me that she'd been sniffing herbs since birth, had never tampered with patriarchal medicine and was therefore impervious to any form of cancer. She was safe. 'This is the legacy of your marriage,' she said sagely, and got up to go. Clearly, it served me right.

The advocates of alternative therapy rose up in droves, delivering advice from a safe distance. Don't have surgery. Don't pollute yourself with chemicals. Ring up the Bristol Cancer Help Centre. Charge yourself with healing energy. Try the Gentle Touch. No one explained what that was. Above all else, DIET. These women recommended bibliographies of possibility. With one voice hospitals and all their works were universally denounced. My illness was due to a lack of harmonious equilibrium in my body, mind and spirit, moral failure, collaboration with men, sexual uncleanliness, meat, heterosexual fornication on a grand scale, which I must have gone in for in the 1960s, not having children, nasty lesbian practices such as dirty fingernails in the vagina, advanced intellectualism which had caused me to lose touch with my body, or – fantastically – the onset of AIDS. I was responsible for having cancer. I could therefore undo the illness myself by positive thinking and a lot of righteous, puritan herbal potions. I am not inventing any of this. I stopped going to the Women's Centre.

One woman sent me an issue of the journal produced by the Bristol Cancer Centre (Winter 1985/1986, Number 4). I am sure that she meant well. The world is full of tearful faces and wrecked lives that have resulted from well-meaning actions. This magazine is appropriately called *Turning Point*. I looked suspiciously at the articles: 'The Meaning of Illness', 'Forgiveness', 'How shall I live?', 'Confessions of a Bristol Dieter'. The cover was in peaceful green with one lone figure of uncertain sex confronting a flat, shining ocean. It also represented what my Catholic aunt calls a 'Jesus sky': a great shimmering disc transfigured by a radiant vortex forming the background to a miraculous superman ascension, or indicating the approach of angels in religious paintings, generally distinguished by their gruesome colours and bad taste. The message on the cover of this magazine was an old one which I had learned from various forms of christianity: that illness and sin are bound together, that we are victims of disease through our own most grievous fault, and that we are therefore desperately in need of forgiveness. If we are ill we have done wrong. I put the magazine down carefully and washed my hands.

My whole life is bound up with the worship of the written word. I read. I write. For me these two procedures are closely intertwined. A woman I once admired entitled her doctoral dissertation 'The Act of Reading', a title which reflected some of the peculiar eroticism I have always experienced in the process. The capacity to read is infinitely precious to me. Now that I was ill I could no longer read. Words, all words, lost their meanings. This has been my experience of the fear of death. I lost all grasp on meaning.

I have always had a peculiar and powerful sense of God. I perceive God as an intimate antagonist, and as a vast, empty chasm, a monstrous non-being whose jaws of unmeaning perpetually threaten the world. God is formidably present in absence, menacingly close. God is the word, present in the word, yet coded, like a hieroglyph. Islam teaches that God is as far as the stars and as close as the pulse of your jugular vein. This has always been true for me. I have very little apprehension of God's love. For me, our pendant world spins forever in the void. This vision is unchristian and horrifying. It is probably heretical. But it is neither smug nor complacent.

When I turned to face my own death, the fragility, not of my own physical existence but of the reasons why I continued to exist at all, rushed to meet me. I knew that I would simply cease to be. I saw Death at last, as the place where God-is-Not. God vanishes, even as the arbiter of unmeaning, and certainly as the healing word. I knew myself to be utterly forsaken. Death is the end of subjective, perceiving consciousness, the end of ourselves as the interpreters of our own lives. And the awareness of what that knowledge implied immediately engulfed me. I looked out at the rows of either cruel or anxiously loving faces before me and knew that neither their lives nor mine had any value or meaning. I sank into a long howl of grief and fear and an absolute, unreachable loneliness. I was utterly without resources. But when I see my death again, as I am waiting to do, it will be to recognise a landscape I already know, to step through a familiar door.

All colour, all purpose had gone. Instead I heard one long scream of pain, an inarticulate shrieking from all the world. My surroundings hung like a tapestry before me. A gap now stretched between reality and the thinking, breathing body I knew to be my own, which no longer possessed the capacity to read or write. And yet it was precisely this loss that I was able to articulate. On 30 April 1986 I wrote this in the Blue Book:

> Alone. Near 10 pm, at home. The first warm nights. I put out the geraniums. The nuns remember me. Not days in which to contemplate the dark. The American raid on Libya, plunging the world closer to war. The giant cloud of radioactive dust from Chernobyl drifting across Europe. From a core of pain I lose my grip on the two things I hold, my writing, my reading. God as faceless. The unspeaking word.
>
> Amazed I am to watch my pen making words. Crossing the page.

On Thursday 17 April 1986, during the week of the American raid on Libya, I was admitted to hospital. My lover, A., who looked as pale, frightened and tearful as I did, came with me. Once I am inside a hospital I no longer even pretend to be brave. On the assumption that once you have actually had the plastic label affixed to your wrist further resistance is useless, I simply subside into a pond of tears. I was weeping miserably over the young woman in pathology when A. was startled by another of the lesbian women in our community, who appeared in the corridor. This was Clare, dressed up as an occupational therapist.

'What are you doing here?' A. demanded hysterically.

'I'm a famous brain surgeon,' said Clare.

A. burst into tears.

When I came round from the anaesthetic later that afternoon Clare had left me a note, simply telling me where I could find her in the hospital. She wrote at the bottom: 'Lots of Love. Lots of Strength. Clare.' I have kept that note ever since.

Two women stayed with me all that day on Ward 1. One of them was A. and the other was a woman named Jill. Ward 1 is the emergency gynaecological ward. Many of the women come in on their backs, collapsed and battered by pain and fear. Sometimes they are weeping and screaming. The abortions often end up next to the miscarriages. Most of the time no one knows what has gone wrong. Very few women ever sleep on this ward. The drama continues day and night. It is a suspended, isolated world. The nurses who work there are frighteningly over-worked and wickedly underpaid. They thankfully abandoned me to Jill and A., who sat beside me in the noisy white world all day.

Unfortunately I have an astonishing resistance to anaesthetic. I place great value upon the conscious, thinking mind; the mind that reasons, judges and remembers. It is this mind which shapes my writing. It is almost impossible to subdue. I saw the pre-operation room where they deliver the anaesthetic with the kind of lurid clarity usually associated with hallucinations. It was painted green and decorated with shining metal pans. The theatre staff wore green – green robes, green masks. The operating theatre was being scrubbed down with a machine which steamed and roared. I saw the great glass circles in the green folding doors misting over.

Doctors now believe that it is important to explain everything that they are about to do to the patient several times over. David Barlow appeared in the middle of my green hallucination, lowered his green mask and began to explain his explanations. My last memory is of clutching his arm savagely in the hope of remaining conscious, and being prised off by one of the nurses.

A cone biopsy removes the centre of tissue in the neck of the womb. It is like cutting the core from an apple. And it hurts. I was left in neces-sary pain, feeling that my body had been cut and torn by strangers and knowing that a laboratory technician would simply analyse tissue belong to PATRICIA DUNCKER: FEMALE, AGED 34, No. 889691, with professional indifference. That piece of bloody tissue contained my life.

I waited in pain for a week. During that time I tried to paste a patchwork of meaning over my blank world. I was in hospital for only two days. I was sanely brave in front of visitors, even taught my students, and tried not to hurl my lover into the void I inhabited. But she was not deceived. My attention, usually fixed upon her, was elsewhere. David Barlow rang me on Friday morning, 25 April 1986, with his version of the good news. The cancer was not yet invasive, but it had indeed spread up the cervical canal. As I had been perfectly and unhesitatingly clear that I never wanted children, he recommended a total abdominal hysterectomy, leaving the ovaries behind.

I went away to a bookshop and bought a pink floral book on hysterectomy.

This book was awarded a pink rosette by the Family Planning Association and was entitled *Hysterectomy: What it is and How to Cope with it Successfully* (Sheldon Press, 1986). The author, Suzie Hayman, was a journalist and she had had a hysterectomy. Glowing with the ideology of patient-power, she wrote the book from the patient's perspective and assumed that every woman is heterosexual and living with her male partner. The book opens with the following sweeping claim. 'The feelings a woman has for her womb are quite unlike the relationship she has with any other part of her body.' There then follow several pages of fairly sensible thoughts on menstruation, bearing children, femininity and the attitudes of male doctors.

I have examined the statement which opens this book both before and after my hysterectomy. I have reflected on it again, 10 years on, and I find that what the author says is not true. After my operation I had a long purple scar across my lower abdomen, torn, bruised muscles, and I could no longer menstruate. I was desperately afraid and distressed at what had happened to me. I grieved for the loss of my womb. Then I forgot all about it. I grieved, no more, no less that I would have done if I had lost several yards of intestine or my big toe. I had already refused to become what Suzie Hayman defines as a woman. According to her, a woman marries, has children, centres her identity on her relationships to men and servicing other people. My life was with other women and with words. What was at stake for me was that life itself.

I was given some unintentional, but very welcome support from a friend. Mardi, then 89 years old, had also had a hysterectomy:

'Don't worry, my dear,' she said airily, dismissing cancer and all its works, 'they take it all away and then you won't have any more problems.'

'How did you feel?' I asked.

'Goodness,' said Mardi, 'it was over 50 years ago. And I haven't thought about it from that day to this.'

I knew only one other lesbian who had had a hysterectomy, Sheila S. I contacted her somewhat late in the day. I have always found it difficult to ask other women for help. Women usually offer help, we don't need it ourselves. This is a fault. We should be brave enough to ask. Without Sheila's story of how she felt, what she had feared, how it was for her, I would have approached my operation with considerably more apprehension and fear. She was funny, warm, supportive, loving. I owe her that love.

A smokescreen of sensible reassurance fluttered up from Suzie Hayman's pages whenever the question of renewed heterosexual sex reared its purple head. I had a lot of doubts about sex and didn't dare ask Mardi, who might also have dismissed the subject to the era of 50 years before. I asked Sheila S. if I would ever be able to make love again.

'Oh yes,' she said, 'it's very little different.' And she went off into frank and comforting explicit detail. 'But no sex for six weeks,' she said firmly, then added, 'Actually, you won't feel like it.'

In fact, I did. Never in all my life have I been so desperate for the touch of a woman's hand and a loving caress. When I returned from the hospital for the second time it was too late. My lover had abandoned me in the existential void into which I had retreated. When I stretched out my arms in sadness and despair, she had already gone.

But she came with me on 6 May 1986, when I went back to the hospital. Men, even the male doctors, are not altogether welcome on

Ward 1. A working-class woman named Suzette was in the bed next to me. She was an emergency admission with an ectopic pregnancy. She had been taking the Pill. But she had been eight weeks' pregnant and she had nearly died. As soon as she was conscious again she rose up out of the anaesthetic and screeched at her boyfriend, who had taken considerable trouble to turn up looking like a young Robert Redford:

'You did this to me! You did it!' with pure venom, hatred and considerable volume. We all looked sorrowful and none of the nurses disagreed. Men and the whole apparatus of heterosexuality and reproduction are usually responsible for all the pain, mess and horror in a gynaecological ward. The two other women in my section, Fereshteh and Elyse, were both having further operations as a result of botched sterilisations done years before. We were all there, either because we were, or because we had been, heterosexual.

Beware, in hospitals, of assuming that the apparently unconscious cannot hear you. As I lay, submerged in white on the end of the drip after my first operation, I heard another woman speaking about me. She was married and had two children. Her husband had abandoned her and had taken up with a sequence of teenage girls. She had read the notes at the bottom of my bed.

'She's got cancer. You know, in the womb. You get it from sex. Poor thing. No man's worth that.'

I agree.

I have said that the world became blank for me: in fact, it became white. White, colourless, meaningless. And it was pain which coloured the tapestry again. Pain, so utterly real, consuming, absorbing, close; pain became the lover's touch. It blossomed in the night. Pain and passion are often associated. They are both subjective experiences and cannot be measured. Before the operation, David Barlow appeared again in the ward with a further litany of explanations.

'Thursday will be a big day for you,' he said, 'because you'll be getting over your operation. But so far as I'm concerned we won't be any further on until we've analysed that uterus in the lab. So it could be early next week before we know anything.'

This was not comforting, but cancer is not a disease that doctors find comforting either. David Barlow is well known for his kindness, but also for his honesty.

The anaesthetist, forewarned of my ferocious refusal to relinquish consciousness, clarity and daylight, doubled the dose. It had no effect. When we reached the Anaesthetic Room I was wheeled underneath a reproduction of Monet's poppy field.

'Take away the Monet,' I commanded from the trolley.

'Good Heavens,' he cried, peering into my face, 'you're all there.'

I rose up from the slab in rage and fear. A struggle ensued and my spectacularly bruised arm was one of the sights on Ward 1 during the following week.

The reality of a hysterectomy, and indeed of every major operation, is pain; exhaustion, depression and pain. I had a great many visitors. It was kind of them to come. The healthy visit the sick in hospital for many different reasons, but unmistakable on every face was the relief that they were not required to inhabit this white kingdom. This was not true of Sheila S. She came up from London bearing gifts, all of which proved to be essential post-operative equipment. She made herself comfortable beside the bed and looked carefully around the ward as if she were planning to move in. She was not at all alarmed at the sight of so many women reduced, humiliated, helpless and diminished. She had no fear. On every other face I read my own fear.

The community of pain in the ward circled around meals, doctors and the lavatory with a mixture of hilarity and resentment. Nursing is a heroic, filthy profession which consists of dealing with showers of urine, excrement and vomit. One of us thought that she was dying. Another patient summoned Sister O'Leary, who was angular, red-headed.

'Dying? Not on this ward, you don't!' she snapped. 'Have you had your bowels open?'

We were not allowed to be hysterical or constipated, and we were forbidden to die.

I have been criticised, to my face, by many feminists and lesbians who were part of the movement 10 years ago, for refusing to use alternative treatments and for abusing my body with patriarchal pills. In fact, like every sensible person I know, I did and do use many simple herbal medicines: Bach's Rescue Remedy, Arnica for shock, Comfrey Ointment for the wound. I spent hours doing Yoga in the ward before my operation, to general amusement and excitement. I practised my deep breathing exercises while one of the nurses removed my surgical clips. I used the meditation techniques I had been taught to sleep peacefully at night and hold the pain at bay. The attitudes of the women at the hospital to all this was warmly appreciative. They watched, listened and tried the remedies themselves. While I was in hospital the British Medical Association published their notorious report discrediting alternative medicines, homeopathy and acupuncture. They are utterly disconnected from the white world where any form of treatment which could contribute to survival and well-being was welcomed without scruple or hesitation. Sister O'Leary read the label on the bottle of Bach Rescue Remedy. She sniffed the contents.

'You carry on, my love. A few flowers and a bit of brandy won't hurt you. And if it does you good, all the better.'

My own attitude to conventional medicine is ambivalent. I was born and brought up in the West Indies, in a poor country which has been exploited by the capitalist West for centuries. The diseases which killed poor people on that island have long been overcome in the wealthy world: diptheria, tuberculosis, polio, meningitis, yellow fever. Our children died of malnutrition, diarrhoea, dehydration, filth and ignorance. The greatest killer was poverty. In Kingston General Hospital, so my mother tells me, they used to bring tea round in a bucket. A revolution in health care, vaccines, penicillin, basic hygiene, was a matter of life and death. We could not heal ourselves with diets and centring energy. We thanked God for antibiotics.

Western orthodox medicine can, quite simply, save our lives. It can also maim, poison, mutilate and kill. I put my trust in other women. My own GP at that time was a woman. She was pragmatic, matter-of-fact, professional. We had nothing in common and she made it quite clear that she had very little time for lesbians. Like most well-off married women with good jobs she did not appear to understand why anyone would want to live otherwise. Or to think differently. She occasionally came out with some extraordinary and upsetting comments. She was not at all warmly sympathetic in the face of nonsense or hysteria. But she knew me. And she knew at once when she first saw me on 23 January 1986, that there was something seriously wrong with me. I never took David Barlow's advice without going back to her. She may have disagreed with me, but she was on my side.

I was cared for by women. Women talked to me, held me, watched with me, comforted me, fed me and marched me off down to the bathroom. It was the women who did all the dirty work. In that and in every other hospital it was the women who saved lives and made people well. Within the NHS they take care of those who are least able to take care of themselves. They are given neither credit nor money. They deserve the earth.

On Thursday 13 May 1986, sometime late in the afternoon, Mr Barlow galloped into the ward like the cavalry, waving the laboratory report. The cancer was not yet invasive in the womb.

'So the story's over, as far as you're concerned.' He was jubilant. 'This is the end of the line for you. If you've got someone to look after you, you can go home tomorrow.'

I tottered down to the phone and I rang my mother and my lover in delight.

'Oh,' said A., when I announced that I could come home as early next day as she could arrive at the hospital. 'Well, it would be more convenient for me if you came home much later in the day.'

But the hospital needed my bed.

My return home marked the beginning of the deepest loneliness and the most terrible pain I have ever known. Suzie Hayman's pink book contained some wise words on the subject of selfishness and fear. She may only have had men, indeed husbands, in mind, but what she wrote proved to be dangerously true of my woman lover:

> When something strikes at our deepest fears, it is a very common reaction to try and block out the pain by pretending its cause does not actually exist. You may be hurt and confused by everyone's apparent indifference to your sufferings ... As soon as you get home they may be amazed and furious if everything is not back to normal at once. It is unlikely that you really have created a house full of unfeeling monsters. At the root of most of this 'selfishness' is an overwhelming fear.

This is perceptive, intelligent – and quite useless, unless the unfeeling monster concerned absorbs the lesson, confronts her fears and puts some effort into self-discipline and self-control. My lover did indeed react in precisely the manner Hayman describes, but the consequences, because she is a woman, were very different than they would have been had she been a man. When a man turns on a woman, abuses, attacks and abandons her, he is only endorsing and reproducing the structures of misogyny which are the scaffolding of our world, a world from which he benefits and which he has probably helped to build. When a woman does this to another woman, she is destroying a part of herself.

A. went on the offensive. She was unable to sleep, and because she could not sleep then I should not sleep either. She said that she found my body physically disgusting, and recoiled accordingly. She raved at me if I cried. She was appalled by my weakness; and by the fact that the strong woman she had always accused of being too remote had vanished, leaving a heap of battered, weeping flesh behind. She abandoned me, not only day after day, but night after night. She took to dining out, drinking late, going off to every social occasion. She screamed abuse at me, stormed and raged at my inadequacy, denounced me for being a sort of emotional swamp. As I no doubt was, given her anger and rejection. She even accused me of malingering. I hadn't actually had cancer, she shouted. It was all my selfish imagination. I had done it to get attention.

I began to feel that I was going insane. The tenuous, brittle grasp I had on reality became more fragile.

One lesbian in our community, who was herself about to undergo a hysterectomy for her fibroids, told me that she hoped her lover would not look as exhausted as A. had done, implying that it was my fault. The bitterness of this remark has never left my tongue. The woman had imagined A.'s exhaustion was due to her anxious, loving watches at my bedside. I was too weak to shop, clean or even to stand at the stove. But I could have died in a sea of filth and hunger as far as my lover was concerned. She would not forgive me because I did not die. And yet she denied what she was doing, even the reality of her own behaviour proved impossible for her to acknowledge. She claimed either not to have said or done – or to have forgotten events of the previous week.

A. was not constant in her abuse. On rare occasions she was friendly, even affectionate. But if I moved towards her, longing for a sign of her love, she turned on me with a savagery and anger which hurt me more than if she had been an impartial, sadistic torturer. I turned my face to the wall.

But in all this I was not alone. I was not utterly abandoned, betrayed or deserted. In my experience of cancer I discovered again the passionate strength of love one woman can have for another. On Friday 16 May 1986, at around 8 o'clock in the morning, my mother appeared on the doorstep. She did not leave me for two weeks; the sense of her presence and the fact of her continuing love is with me now. She simply took over responsibility for the house, the washing, shopping, cooking, cleaning. She kept the show on the road. She dealt with the telephone, the visitors, flowers. She fed the cat, put out the dustbin, went to the chemist's, locked the doors. She held me when I was in pain, woke with me in the night, comforted my despair, sat peacefully beside me when

I slept, wiped the tears from my eyes. The only sign I ever had of her anxiety, worry and fear was that she lost weight dramatically over the weeks. If she was ever afraid for my life, I never knew. She never spoke of herself. She offered only encouragement and strength, her hand. And she made me understand that love is not something you declare, nor even something you feel, or smugly enjoy; it is something you do for someone else, day after day after day.

She did not come to me simply because she is my mother. She has not always supported me. Over the years our relationship has been angry, bitter, difficult. The reason for this is that I, demanding her love and approval, have always tried to treat her as my mother, upon whom I had an absolute claim. I wanted to be her daughter, not her friend. I wanted her unconditional love. I was not prepared to stomach her criticism, her rationalism and her refusal to endorse my behaviour if her judgement led her to think differently. I refused what she offered to me, which was the constructive, critical support one woman can offer to another woman she loves. She is not, and never will be, easy to know. She is silent, opaque, ferociously independent, eccentric and strange. She regards the material desires of those that have and the passions which shape the kingdom of this world with an informed contempt. She is an ascetic; her judgements are never voiced. Through all the years we were together as mother and daughter, I never understood her values, nor her love. I do now.

When my mother had to leave me and return to her work in London, other women, lesbians and married women, took her place. They came armed with food, they sent cards and flowers, they took me out in their cars to see the coming spring, they wrote, they rang up. I remember each occasion and each one of them. I even had two men – the only two I knew well – who lined up as supporters. We had cooperative driving sessions. One of them used to haul up the handbrake when I was too weak to lift it off the floor of the car. They both came to cook, and they both washed up without expecting universal admiration and thanks. I shall remember every gesture, every word of kindness. And I kept all the cards.

But those who were not with me were against me, and that too I shall never forget.

My lover had asked my mother to come. I think it is important to make this clear in the light of what subsequently happened. My mother was careful to steer round A. and never to confront her about her rages, her appalling behaviour and her screaming abuse. My mother treated my lover as she had always done, with great courtesy and caution. She was usually adept at manouevring round the edges of A.'s temper. But at last this proved impossible to do. A. perceived my mother's very competence and support which was also offered to her, as a gratuitous insult. She accused my mother of taking over the house, of going out to Tesco's without adequate consultation, of buying tomatoes, and, inter-estingly, of reducing herself to a serf. My mother pointed out to me that A. had actually eaten the offending tomatoes. And presumably only serfs bothered to do a little cooking and cleaning. Then, hysterically, shining with health and strength, A. claimed that she was ill, frail, weak, vulnerable. This was odd, but it had its own mad logic. She claimed to be all the things I was. Her violence did me enormous damage. I sank into a terrible corrosive depression. There was no way of stopping her. She wanted me out of the house. She wanted me out of her sight. She wanted me removed to London. I felt too weak to move. And so she spoke to Sheila S. on the telephone. Sheila, drawing on her own experience of hysterectomy, sensibly pointed out that A. was the one who was able to move. 'Why don't you live somewhere else?' she asked. A. came downstairs, amazed. 'She suggested that I should move out. That had never occurred to me.' My mother and I looked at each other. It had never occurred to us either, because the point of the exercise had so clearly been to drive me out of the house.

– Where is God?
– In us, or nowhere.
On Saturday 17 May 1986 I wrote in the Blue Book:

One of the Great Christian Lies. That suffering and fear are powerful enriching experiences. The human spirit diminishes, shrivels, withers into demoralised misery. I feel less human, less strong.

But I had begun to read again. On Thursday 3 June 1986 I wrote, 'Salvation lies in the Book. All Books.' And it was because I had learned to read and write again that I survived.

The doctors forbade me to move for two months. At 11.30 on the night which marked the passing of the forbidden months I set sail for France. During that time abroad I gnawed and chewed at what had happened between myself and the woman I had so passionately loved.

In Paris on Thursday 10 July 1986, I spent the afternoon in the laundrette:

The laverie in the rue St. Ambroise. Around 11.20. Funny how courageous and powerful I feel at having more or less gained control of the washing machine in French. It is scrupulously clean. With sinister neat instructions in great diagrams across the walls. No money will be reimbursed if the machine doesn't work … I am 35 … The moment to look both ways. There is a strong voice in me which moves me so much I want to cry, break down and weep, even here in the middle of the laundrette – that says 'Have done, seek silence. Write.' But I still love A. I was not detached. I am still in love with her – as much as I have always been. It is just that now I see her entire – as I had refused to do. See her also as she is, egotistical, selfish, malicious, confused, unhappy, unstable.

If only she would really work on her difficulties – rather than shore up her ego by paying Clare large sums of money to stick needles into her feet and come out with cryptic utterances like 'You're blocked between water and metal.' Whatever that means.

Even in our two conversations on the subject James spoke up for her so warmly. Pointed out the ways in which – however insanely cruel she may have seemed – she was only reacting to the fact that by becoming so critically ill I had utterly changed the rules of the relationship and had suddenly demanded something of her – it makes me sound like the Lord, flattening Job out of the whirlwind. But it's true that I never tried to demand anything of her. Tried hard because I'd seen what happened to anyone who did. They were either savaged, neglected or ignored. And she turned on me when I had the nerve to develop cancer and say 'I need you now'...

Doing the laundry is actually a very peaceful thing to do. The world turns symbolically before you at the touch of a button. Without your doing. A steady hum in the driers with the constant click of buttons against metal. I have lost the thread ...

The habit of self-analysis, self-criticism, self-questioning is crucial for any writer. Without it we dissolve ever more rapidly into pompous sententiousness. I struggled to interrogate myself in the Blue Book. And I perceived however dimly, that the death of love in my own life was bound up with the retreat from God. On Bastille Day, Monday 14 July 1986, I did something quite uncharacteristic: I went out to watch the military parade passing down the Champs Elysées. I wrote:

The parade was rather extraordinary, ornamental soldiers wearing metal and feathers, followed by row after row of sinister khaki-green coloured armoured cars, tanks, missile-launchers with very slender pointed missiles. The Foreign Legion got a warm round of applause, as did the Sapeurs, Pompiers de Paris, who came at the end. But the crowd did become baffled and quiet as the tanks passed ... I watched at last without fear. I have been gone two weeks and feel no nearer a decision. All I see is a huge and fearful emptiness. This is partly because I am so far from my work. So bereft of my context of living. So demoralised by my mutilated stomach, my sense of my own powerlessness. So alienated from my community.

But in fact I was then very near to the decision I had to make. I had begun to look outwards, to do the laundry myself, to judge the world and to look, unafraid, at the world preparing for war.

I went to Paris to see another woman who had cancer, breast cancer. She had spent a whole year in pain, having radiotherapy and chemotherapy. She lived alone. On 9 June 1986 she had written to me. Here is that letter in its entirety. When I first read this letter I burst into tears:

> *Dear Patricia*
>
> *Colin just phoned – and said that you had to go through an operation because of a cancer problem recently. Though I know they fix you straight for another forty years, I am sorry all the same – such a nuisance. Now I am glad I can tell for once 'Look at me' – I hope you are not too exhausted – you must be careful in the forthcoming months. Don't start working in a neurotic way, like so many 'miraculés de cancer' do.*
>
> *Speaking of miraculés de la medicine moderne: I don't suggest that we start a club of narrow escapes or whatever. In my opinion <u>they</u> will have to start a club, the people who never had cancer. Such a minority.*
>
> *I hope you are well looked after – that you choose the very best hospital and the most efficient doctors. Colin said you had not to go through chemotherapy and radiotherapy. Thank Goodness for that! At least some side-effects will be spared to you. As for the side-effects which won't be spared, let us hope they will be light. I'm particularly thinking of psychological effects. You are a strong woman, Patricia, and though a woman always resents a loss of that kind we can cope, can't we? I am so accustomed to the new shape of my breast now, that I just can't imagine that it used to be different.*
>
> *Hear-say-radio may have let you know already that my application to a permanent fellowship was successful. There is a life after cancer, indeed, and a lovely one.*

Take care of yourself. Be good. Rest plenty. A deck chair in the garden and the complete works of Dorothy Sayers, that's my prescription. And a lot of laughs. Remember: a big laugh thrice a day keeps worries away (and people with no sense of humour as well, which is a blessing).
Lots of Love (and to A.)
Michèle

On Sunday 20 July 1986 we went out to talk and to eat. This is what I wrote two days later, on Tuesday 22 July 1986:

That night I had supper with Michèle at Chez Jenny, the brasserie at République which is famous for its sauerkraut. We sat in the window, there were tables outside, catching a faint draught. It is not all negative, says Michèle. She finds herself able to be at once more charming and able to speak up for herself. Charming to men, that is. Feminism, she says, held her back. She comes over as odd, someone self-contained by force. In her flat she read me the substance of her forthcoming interview with Australian radio. It was a philosophical autobiography, with some very witty anecdotes.

I told Michèle what had happened. She was not surprised. It is the norm for those who are closest to turn most savagely against the person who is ill. One of the women having chemotherapy described it as the *Descente dans l'enfer*. I understood. And Michèle had had friends to be with her, to hold her hands. She understood the weakness, how humiliated, afraid, demoralised we were. She said 'Yes, it does hang – Damocles' sword – over us now, but no more than it has always done over everyone else. We see, simply, what is there. It is a privileged vision to have.' And, most perceptively, she saw that I, as the stronger one, had shifted the terms of the game. And had demanded the love, attention, commitment and support which I had always given before. But how could I have chosen not to do so? A. had asked and asked, and I had given. Oh, reason not the need. Well, I should have reasoned. Every drop.

While I was in France my lover wrote to me in a brief and passing moment when she realised who she was and what she had done. She wrote on 10 July 1986:

> I think I'm very self-repressed, and intend to give myself more space for relaxing and enjoying myself. And then perhaps I shall stop blaming others, nearest and dearest, you, for feeling restricted. I do feel most terribly trapped inside some self-imposed shell, out of which I should like some help getting. Does this make sense?...
>
> Clare said just before I left that she thought I had some enormous block, an emotional/physiological block which recurs and incapacitates me.
>
> I am very sorry for not having been the source of solid comfort and support you have justly wanted to be able to expect. I don't know what happened, but must, I think, find out. I don't think of myself as mean and ungenerous. But that is certainly how I have been. Can you forgive it? I know it's a lot to ask in return for my quite inappropriate resistance and withdrawal. I don't understand it at all.

There was a complete disjunction between this open apology and what had actually happened, which I found and still do find particularly disquieting. When I was weak and frightened she set out to bully, persecute and destroy. It was as if someone who had tried to hack you to death suddenly apologised for bruising your finger. But it was better than nothing. I went back, intending to work for reconciliation. I found her waiting, like a pack of wolves.

We are, as women, rewarded for lying, for deceiving ourselves and deceiving each other. The lying built into lesbianism is the pressure to deny who we are, and what we are to each other. It was easy for my lover to retreat into a wine barrel of lies. So far as the heterosexual world was concerned, we counted for nothing, scarcely existed other than as an occasional pinch of spicy gossip. She rightly concluded that the only place where she had to maintain an aggressively high profile was within the groups of lesbians where we had found our company, our political life and our friends. If she could not put herself unequivocally beyond reproach, then she could at least appear powerful and unpleasant enough to avoid repercussions. For this was the place where she could justly claim support. In the straight world she was on her own, and she knew it. It was therefore necessary for her to sever my fragile links with the lesbian community, to destroy my network of friends and my support, in order to bolster her own. She pounced on the telephone like a starving bear, greeting every caller with a remorseless, loud affability. This volley of good nature was punctuated by machine-gun laughter. I found her telephone technique particularly nasty, as the kind words to the absent speaker were followed moments later, by venom and vindictiveness towards me. She conducted a war, unheard, malicious, unseen. During the last days I was driven out of the house for weeks on end, living in sleeping bags, in a friend's studio, in my mother's house, in the back of my car, on the road.

I am not, and never have been, a passive masochist. As soon as I had the strength to do so I fought back. I gave A. a taste of all the venomous abuse and contempt which she had meted out to me, measure still for measure. But this was not worth the trouble. She loved the whole transaction, sleek, trim, fit, glowing with health and smug sadism, at last she had what she had wanted all along: a real fight. I do not share her professional commitment to malice. I could not live on those terms. Yet I was deeply shaken by the truth of something she had said during the worst of the May days: 'I was like this all along. And you just never noticed.' In fact, I *had* noticed. But I had a naïve and arrogant faith in the strength of love to forgive and transform. What I had done was excuse and condone. And I had done this for the very worst of reasons. I took responsibility for my lover in the way that women do for their appalling husbands and their atrocious, spoiled children. Where she was selfish, rude, mean or unkind I tried to mend the breach, stitching up the rent with good will, pasting the splintered tempers back together again. I was wrong to do this. It was my attempt to control her and the anger between us.

'I feel that nothing I give will ever be enough,' wailed A., and therefore decided to give nothing at all.

And yet I loved her because she was my apparent opposite. She dealt in abstract theory; I dealt in the particulars of daily life. Her philosophy moved outwards towards a total theory of being. I saw single people in unique situations. She advocated unlimited speculation. I believed in certainties of my own making. But when I turned to face illness and death we discovered that I was the rationalist, the atheist, a recluse in the desert; my lover needed the trivial, the particularity of this world, and a night out drinking to ward off approaching ghosts. 'I can't live like this,' she shrieked, during the weeks of waiting, 'right on the edge of Apocalypse. I can't stand it. I can't take it.'

Well, I think we have to, and most of the time, I can.

Even at the beginning the idea of the curse was never a joke. We planned to enact a ritual curse, to end my connection with this woman forever. Two members of a group with which I was involved, the Women's Theology Seminar, hatched the plot together. Kate had been doing some research on classical Egyptian curses. She told Anne what to do. Anne, however, began to invent freely, though to what extent this altered the effect of the original recipe, we shall never know. Anne was the other woman who saved my life. She is extraordinary, gifted, powerful. Ten years on, we are still together. Our lives have altered dramatically since the days when we built the curse, but I can see no shadow of any parting between us. Without her, I would not have survived. Without her, I could not go on.

This was the curse:

'Steal a pot. Something she's touched and owned. Something she's had a long time. Write her name on it. Burn the herbs of bitterness within it. Then, when the moment is right, speak the curse and smash the pot.'

It was an extraordinarily simple symbolic action; a straightforward gesture, to send back all the cruelty and pain she had handed out to me, and to set me free to live my own life again. A woman's revenge always captures the imagination. Her many revenges haunted me: Verdi's Azucena, with her right hand clasped forever, avenging her mother's destruction; Medea, smiling, the shirt of Nessus folded in her hands; Clytemnestra, claiming her husband's life in return for that of her daughter, staging her revenge with ritual and guile. The wrongs against these women were done openly by men, but their revenge was planned in secret, achieved through cunning, trickery, witchcraft.

At first, I hesitated. In Jamaica people actually die from the vindictive ingenuity of their neighbours. British colonial law could not deal with obeah, and operated with a wonderful species of double-think. Obeah did not exist. It was also banned. My unfortunate father was a local magistrate and therefore often forced to listen to accusations of sorcery, obeah, magic, the effectiveness of which was indubitable, but naturally impossible to prove. I do not know whether I believe in Obeah: nevertheless, I hesitated. However, what happened during the last days was violent and extraordinary. And changed my mind.

Her behaviour was not sane. She was a woman obsessed. The long, shrieking phone calls reached a hysterical pitch. The phone bill reached £179. She began to follow me around the house, sometimes insinuating, sometimes abusive, demanding that I should listen to her diatribes. I did a very simple, cruel thing: I refused to speak. I no longer had anything to say. Nor was I willing to listen to her lies. When she began to scream I walked out of the room. Sometimes she pursued me, shouting. Once, and only once, she struck me. My silence increased the frenzy of her performance, as it was intended to do. For this was part of my revenge. In May and June I had been too weak to walk. By September I could simply stride out of the house. But the cost proved too great in the flesh.

With their own uncanny sense of the symbolic, my internal wounds ceased to heal. This was not surprising. I was exhausted and on edge. When I slept she came home in the early hours, turned on all the lights and crashed up the stairs. The cat and I watched in the darkness until the house was silent. He slept in the daytime. I was worn to a wretched state of near hysteria.

The symptoms were those that had first indicated that the cancer was within me. Pain. I trailed wretchedly back to my doctor. Once you have had cancer, any subsequent ailment is suspected of being another cancer. My doctor set her mouth and did all the usual tests. She looked grim. I looked upset, but with weary self-control I managed not to cry. The first smear collapsed. The cells were exposed for too long in the air and caved in. I sympathised with the cells. We did all the tests again. And this time, facing the remote but possible eventuality of radio-therapy and a prolonged, painful illness, I sank into an absolute despair. My recovery was a sick joke. It was as if God had given me back my life only to take away all the things that had made it worth the living. I no longer had a home, a political community or someone to love. If I could neither read nor write again I chose to die. And so I no longer bothered either with existential questions or with God. I simply went to bed, exhausted, and swallowed every pill I could lay my hands upon.

I am not normally suicidal, on account of my political convictions. Think how many lesbian tales end with the heroines doomed, damned and dead. This alone should fill us with the savage tenacity to live, love, fight on. They want us dead. We should never give in. If argued into a corner from which I am required to produce a moral absolute, I would probably admit that our lives are not ours to take. Halfway through the second bottle of pills I realised what I was doing, staggered downstairs and rang my mother. But I found myself unable to say that I was halfway through taking an overdose. It sounded too out of character, and frankly bizarre. Instead I wept piteously and managed to stutter, 'There isn't even anyone here to make me a cup of tea.' My mother caught the next train.

By the time she arrived I was very ill indeed. And I don't remember the rest of that night at all clearly. I can just remember Anne's face, completely calm, close to my own. Then I cannot remember anything until morning, when I awoke with a volcanic headache and saw my mother standing beside me with the prophetic cup of tea.

Later I confessed to my doctor that I had swallowed all the sleeping pills. 'Oh, did you? And what were you taking?' She looked savagely into the file, saw the names of the drugs and slammed the file shut, her prescription pad beneath it. 'That's the last lot of pills you ever get from me,' she snapped. She was quite right.

In fact the cancer tests were clear. Once more on the slab at the hospital I peered back up at the white coat, white hair and young face of David Barlow. 'You're not healing,' he said, 'get some rest.' 'Well, things are very difficult…' I muttered unintelligibly. But Anne, angered to the limit of her loyalty and love, had begun the curse.

I stole the pot which had been on the windowsill of the dark house by the canal where A. had lived when I first knew her, and Anne began to burn the herbs of bitterness: wormwood, hyssop, yarrow, rue and hemlock, the philosopher's poison herb. Anne's anger grew directly from her love for me. Looking back, touching the roots of my magic childhood, I know that what we did was terrifying. We reversed A.'s evil, but we gave it shape and potency, we articulated her malicious sadism into a refined and sharpened force. Step by step and week by week, we built the curse.

On the night of the dark moon we two slid silent into the back garden where we had built a spiral terrace of circular bricks. The spiral is the symbol of eternity, the sign of the dragon, particularly associated in ancient mythology with women's power. We placed the pot, black with burnt herbs and incense, sandalwood, frankincense, sweet herbs, at the core of the spiral and burned A.'s image and her hair. Then we broke the spiral, took the four bricks from the centre and carried them to the dark gardens of the college where A. worked. It was as if we had carried a corpse in the back of the car. We were quite silent, quite mad. I laid the four bricks near a pine tree by the gate, spoke the curse and smashed the pot. It is a strange and hideous sound, a single explosion, with no echo. The others had waited in the car. As I stepped out of the darkness we knew that I was free and that her power over me was broken for ever.

My life has been a sequence of radical shifts, sudden and dramatic change. There has been very little continuity. I have lived in different countries, counted more homes than years, broken irrevocably with the lovers who have never been my friends. I never have been, and never will be rich, and if I have not always been warm, I have at least always had something to eat and somewhere to sleep. That is enough. I take the responsibility for who I am and what I have done. I do not believe that we should shift the blame for who we are onto our parents, our family histories, our lovers and friends, our economic circumstances. But we should still judge ourselves and each other with uncompromising clarity and infinite compassion. Unless we judge, we cannot forgive. But we must know the precise cost of our loss, the exact measure of the violence against us. I have told you a story of love, and the betrayal of love. When I was ill I was surrounded by Job's Comforters, confused, well-meaning women, emotional dishonesty, sadistic malice and real empowering love. I have learned anew the uses of anger. Anger is a cathartic force. We should know how to curse and to bless.

My lover may have imagined herself restricted and repressed, but in fact she unleashed every whim, mood, desire and rage whenever she liked. Her self-imposed shell does, I am sure, exist at a very deep level, but I saw no signs of discipline or containment of any kind in her daily behaviour. When I challenged this she simply said that it was not in her power to amend it. I remembered Iago: 'Virtue? A fig! tis in ourselves, that we are thus, or thus: our bodies are gardens, to the which our wills are gardeners, so that if we will plant nettles, or sow lettuce, set hyssop, and weed up thyme … why, the power and corrigible authority of this, lies in our wills.' Well, my lover was interested in gardening, but was never able to proceed beyond an attentive neglect; she planted both nettles and lettuce, and let them both run to seed.

The moment of my understanding that even our friendship was over came when I started work again. I was teaching a Romantics Summer School in the Lake District. The hotel staff where we stayed were all smiles to see me.

'We've put you back in room 165,' the hotel clerk said sweetly, 'last April you said how much you liked that room.' This was the room where I first heard from my doctor that the cancer tests had been positive, that I was to cancel all my plans and come straight back. The tall white man was waiting for me.

When I walked into that room I walked straight into what I had left there, a thick slab of fear, the fear of death. I rang my lover on the evening of Saturday 9 August 1986. I was in tears.

'What have you done?' I cried.

I felt those four months clinging against me, and the emptiness of the mountains outside. She did not know, so she said, she had no idea. But somehow, her love, the great love of which she had boasted, had simply gone. As soon as I became ill her love had gone.

'And it just hasn't come back,' so she said to me. She was distant, brutal and cold. At that I put down the phone and sobbed uncontrollably for hours.

But then something savage and hard grew inside me. For I knew that her obsession had gained its own momentum. She was enthralled by her power over me, and her own capacity to destroy. I never really spoke to her again.

I received very little support from the lesbians in my community when my lover turned against me. I later discovered that she had in fact let it be known that I did not want to see anyone and had shut myself up in the moated grange. She then behaved as if I had ceased to exist. Only two other lesbians took the trouble to look for me and to ask me what had happened. My lover presented herself as the injured party, appeared drunk at her feminist theory group, performed like an acrobat on speed, and took up neurotic smoking to indicate her state of extreme distress. No one apparently bothered to wonder why someone who had endured two operations for cancer and a hysterectomy would want to destroy her entire life, reject her lover, sell her house, give up her paid work, and depart into the void.

There are three central reasons for this. I am not an unapproachable person, but I never ask for help. I find it very difficult to confide in other people. No one would have assumed that I needed help, as I had never needed it before. We had been happy together and demonstrably enjoyed one another's company. For three years we had been at seminars, discussion groups, discos, punting trips, demonstrations, and put on something of a double act. We often disagreed in public, but we backed each other up. There was no party line, but visible mutual support. One of the two women who came to find me pointed out that it had been very important for her to believe that we were happy. We represented what does, unfortunately, sound like a rosary of Victorian values: stability, loyalty, integrity, love and trust. No one wanted to watch the painful destruction of something which they had valued and in which they had believed. As if to prove the point, the woman who had come to say these things never came again.

The third reason is more sinister. Pain, illness and death are our travelling companions. Not all of us will live to be spry old dykes at 80, playing croquet, swigging gin and diverting younger lesbians with entertaining stories of the good old days. Cruelty, violence and distress have tentacles which implicate us if we know what is happening. It is better not to know.

And so I lost all sense of a social context or of a community into which I had put a good deal of time and energy. My absence at every event was noted, as was the reason – namely that my lover dominated every gathering in order to shut me out. She herself recognised that she was doing this, for it was quite deliberate. One evening towards the end she left me a note on the kitchen table pointing out that she would be away and that I was therefore free to go to the lesbian social gathering. But by then I had no wish even to see the women who had abandoned me when I needed them. I tell you this to make a simple point: that when we rely solely on good will to hold a community together, we connive in the rule of the strongest and loudest and the silencing of the weak. The custom and practice which is the norm in the outside world will hold sway over us.

The project of lesbian ethics and a lesbian community which can embrace all the political diversity of sexual practice within lesbian love seems a faint, hopeless dream. I am not optimistic. For when I was abandoned, cornered and in despair, the people who stayed beside me and went the second mile, long after the drama of hospitals and biopsies was over, through the terrible slow haul of convalescence, the depression of a very slow recovery, constantly sabotaged and jeopardised by my lover's irresponsibility and malice, were not lesbians and had no visible vested interest in lesbian politics. The people to whom I owe my life are Anne Jacobs, whom I had known then for barely three years through the Women's Theology Seminar, now spectacularly defunct; James Read, one of my oldest friends, who now lives in France; and my mother. When I look coldly at the reasons for this I see two things. First, that these were the people who loved me, whatever their reasons, and secondly, that they were not afraid of my lover's bad temper, dreadful behaviour and sharp tongue because they did not have to work with her, encounter her day after day. They had nothing to lose.

I dislike confessions. I do not believe that it is either wise or necessary to harangue the world with our agony or our helplessness. But I have been criticised for being too reticent, too enclosed, too opaque, too confused and too difficult to understand. I have never been confused, but I have been silent. To every woman who has accused me of these things, what I have written here is my reply.

My lover is not my enemy. No other woman ever can be. But she will never again be my friend. Love affairs do end, relationships break down, affections change; this is as true of lesbians as of anybody else. But this is not precisely what happened to me. The political and emotional meanings of this betrayal are different. We are a community under threat. We are not secure. The world outside has a vested interest in our disintegration, and our destruction. We are not supported by those who shape their lives around families, marriage, and giving in marriage. Therefore, if we isolate, abandon or neglect any one of our own, for whatever cause, we are taking the knife to ourselves. We must not project our own fears and difficulties onto other women. We must learn to be more tough-minded, more self-critical. We must take responsibility for what we do. We must learn to love one another in more practical, generous ways. We cannot count on anyone else to do that.

The heterosexual world within which we may wish to struggle for a place, a name, a salary, will demand in return that we deny ourselves and each other. Any one of us can attempt that split between a private reality and a public lie. The cost is our integrity, of body and soul. My lover wanted status, authority and power. She cultivated a brash macho swagger in her work and in her manner. She got the part. But it is only a part, a role; and in playing that part we take on the masks of men. It no longer becomes an intellectually incoherent position to mouth feminist theory or lesbian ethics, to stop easily across the peaks of abstraction and yet abandon our lovers when they are too weak to move. This split is characteristic of masculinity; this is the gulf between masculine ideology and the bodies of women, between private cruelty and public respect. But we may all live it successfully for a time – I know I certainly did when I was married. But the price is simple and absolute: at the core of who we are, we cease to be.

Human beings do not necessarily become great-hearted, courageous and noble in the face of catastrophe. They become more visibly, frighteningly, dangerously what they have always been. In the hospital I became a pond of tears, which, in the following months, gradually hardened into a ruthless sea of sharp ice. Nor as we lurch towards our own deaths do we necessarily at last understand the passionate significance of love. We sometimes become locked away from each other for ever, and our great love dies with us.

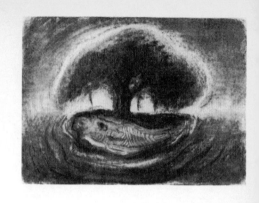

Boadicea

Further Reading

CAROLE COLBOURN

Anne Brontë, *The Tenant of Wildfell Hall* (London: Penguin, 1979). *A classic account of coping with life and adversity.*

Sheila Cassidy, *Audacity to Believe* (London: Darton, Longman & Todd, 1992).

——, *Sharing the Darkness* (London: Darton, Longman and Todd, 1988). *A book born out of the author's work and experience as medical director of St Luke's Hospice.*

Father Francis MacNutt, *Healing* (New York: Bantam, 1977). *A sensible and encouraging approach to a difficult problem.*

Ed Wheat, *Love Life for Every Married Couple* (London: Marshall, 1984). *A biblical study by a psychiatrist who counsels people in crisis.*

John White, *Changing On the Inside* (Guildford: Eagle, 1991). *A practical guide to emotional recovery based broadly on the '12 steps' model used by Alcoholics Anonymous.*

EVELYN DALE

Catallus, 'Poem 51'
Euripides, *The Bacchae*
Susan Hill, *Bird of the Night* (Hamish Hamilton, 1972)
Deborah Hutton, *Vogue Futures* (Ebury, 1996)
Diana Moran, *A More Difficult Exercise* (Bloomsbury, 1989)
Jean Rook, *The Cowardly Lioness* (Sidgwick & Jackson, 1989)
William Shakespeare, *King Lear*
Tom Stoppard, *The Real Inspector Hound* (Faber & Faber, 1968)
Christina Probert, *Vogue Health and Beauty Encyclopaedia* (Hamlyn, 1989)
Tennessee Williams, *A Streetcar Named Desire* (Samuel French, 1953)

DEBBIE DICKINSON

Thomas Moore, *Care of the Soul* (HarperCollins*Publishers*, 1992). *A guide for cultivating depth and sacredness in everyday life. I read this after having written my account for this collection, and felt completely excited by it – so many of the feelings I experienced are articulated wonderfully and eloquently in its pages. Essential reading for anyone who feels an emptiness or confusion about the purpose or point of existence. This book inspires and comforts at the same time, and offers a wealth of insight in a most accessible and poetic fashion.*
Jane Roberts, *Seth: The Nature of Personal Reality* (Bantam Books, 1974)
——, *Seth Speaks* (Bantam Books, 1974). *I love Seth – these books are wonderful, fantastical and believable. Have fun with them.*
Gloria Steinem, *A Book of Self Esteem: Revolution from Within* (Corgi, 1992). *An inspiring and grounded approach to the split between identity and self. A great complement to Thomas Moore's book.*

PATRICIA DUNCKER

When I was ill I couldn't read, words ceased to make sense, so there were no books which I read at the time that were either comforting or useful. But there are two books which have made an enormous difference since then. Primo Levi's novel of Jewish resistance and survival *If Not Now, When?* (Abacus, 1987) has helped me immeasurably over the last years. The savage wisdom which I drew from this book was simple. If you do not fight for yourself no one else will fight for you. The other book which has transformed my memory of cancer is Jane Smiley's novel *A Thousand Acres* (Flamingo, 1992). The character of Rose, who dies of cancer, seemed to me superb, just, terrifying.

MARILYN HACKER

I can't say I consistently sought out books about cancer, or books by people who'd experienced the disease, while undergoing treatment. Sometimes I did; sometimes that was the last subject about which I wished to read. While I was in hospital, I read *Their Ancient Glittering Eyes*, by poet Donald Hall – who is, in fact, a cancer survivor; this is a book, though, about his meetings with poets of an older generation, several of whom lived and worked into their 80s: I needed to read about old poets. A book of Hall's own poems, which did deal with his own (and his wife, poet Jane Kenyon's) experience with cancer, *The Museum of Clear Ideas*, was one I came back to often in the following months. Both of Hall's books were published in the US by Ticknor & Fields. Breast cancer survivor Edith Konecky's novel, *A Place at the Table*, was a book which gave me cheer and courage. (I read this in a Ballantine paperback.)

Long before my illness, I had read Audre Lorde's *The Cancer Journals* and *A Burst of Light* (published by Pandora, 1996) – and these books were a source of strength, perhaps especially because they were already part of my mental background. I would say the same for

Sonny Wainwright's *Stage V: A Journey Through Illness* (Acacia Press). And I would recommend two anthologies of activist essays: *Cancer as a Woman's Issue,* Midge Stocker (ed) (Third Side Press), and *One in Three: Women With Cancer Confront an Epidemic,* Judy Brady (ed) (Cleis Press). And a memoir: *Le Crabe sur la banquette arrière* by Elisabeth Gille (Mercure de France).

I also read a lot of poetry, fiction and essays by writers confronting HIV and AIDS: Thom Gunn's *The Man With Night Sweats* (Faber), Olga Broumas' *Perpetua* (Copper Canyon), Dale Peck's *Martin and John,* Mark Doty's *My Alexandria* (HarperCollins), Tory Dent's *What Silence Equals* (Sheep Meadow) Hervé Guibert's *Le protocole compassionel* and *A l'ami qui ne m'a pas sauvé la vie* (Gallimard).

HILDA RAZ

It seems to me that the literature of witness is little help to us; often the texts depend on accounts of horrors we all experience, not the transforming power of literary texts that can help to make sense of what is an impossible experience to understand fully. The following books helped me:

Oliver Sachs, *A Leg To Stand On* (NY: HarperCollins. rev. ed., 1994). A book by this distinguished writer/physician about his experience with phantom leg syndrome in which his medical colleagues refused to believe.

Susan Sontag, *Illness as Metaphor* (NY: Farrar, Veraus and Giroux, 1978). Though she had cancer, Sontag chose not to speak of her own illness but to analyse cultural attitudes to illness in nineteenth- and twentieth-century Europe and America. She showed me that cancer is, for us, what TB was in nineteenth-century Europe: a disease with moral implications (see Thomas Mann's *The Magic Mountain*, for instance).

Reynolds Price, *A Whole New Life* (Macmillan, 1994). A great writer's experience of cancer of the spine.

Lucy Greeley, *Autobiography of a Face* (NY: HarperCollins, 1995). Her experience of cancer of the jaw.

Thich Nhat Hanh, *The Miracle of Mindfulness: A Manual on Meditation* (Boston: Beacon Press, 1992).

FELLY NKWETO SIMMONDS

Judy Brady (ed.), *One in Three: Women with Cancer Confront an Epidemic* (Pittsburgh and San Francisco: Cleis Press, 1991)

Sandra Butler and Barbara Rosenblum, *Cancer in Two Voices* (San Francisco: Spinsters Ink, 1991)

Erica J. Chopich and Margaret Paul, *Healing Your Aloneness: Finding Love and Wholeness through Your Inner Child* (San Francisco: Harper and Row, 1990)

Stephanie Dworick, *The Intimacy and Solitude Self-Therapy Book* (London: The Women's Press, 1993)

Louise L. Hay, *You Can Heal Your Life* (London: Eden Grove Editions, 1988)

Bell Hooks, *Sisters of the Yam: Black Women and Self-Recovery* (London: Turnaround, 1993)

Harriet Goldhor Lerner, *The Dance of Anger: A Woman's Guide to Changing Patterns of Intimate Relationships* (London: Pandora, 1992)

——, *The Dance of Deception: Pretending and Truth-Telling in Women's Lives* (London: Pandora, 1993)

——, *The Dance of Intimacy: A Woman's Guide to Courageous Acts of Change in Key Relationships* (London: Pandora, 1992)

Audre Lorde, *The Andre Lorde Compendium* (London: Pandora, 1996)

——, *A Burst of Light* (Ithaca, NY: Firebrand, 1988)

——, *The Cancer Journals,* (London: Sheba, 1985)

Evelyn C. White (ed.), *The Black Women's Health Handbook: Speaking for Ourselves* (Seattle: The Seal Press, 1990)

JACKIE STACEY

Books I found useful when I had cancer and chemotherapy include Trish Reynolds' *Your Cancer, Your Life* (Macdonald Optima, 1988) – a good biomedical reference book; Susan Sontag's *Illness as Metaphor* (Penguin, 1978) – a welcome counter to metaphorical interpretations of cancer and other illnesses; Audre Lorde's *The Cancer Journals* (new edition, Pandora, 1996) – a powerful personal narrative with a political edge; Sandra Butler and Barbara Rosenblum's *Cancer in Two Voices* (Spinsters Ink, 1991) – a collaborative journal written by two lesbians who are in a relationship, one of whom is living with/dying of cancer. Some of the 'alternative' accounts offered useful strategies, such as Penny Brohn's *Gentle Giants* – a personal recovery narrative – or her more general *The Bristol Programme* (both Century Publishing, 1987), but these should be read with a critical eye. Finally, and more recently, I found Gillian Rose's *Love's Work* (Chatto and Windus, 1995), a personal and philosophical memoir, quite breathtaking.

Natural Healing for Women
Caring for yourself with herbs, homoeopathy and essential oils
Susan Curtis and Romy Fraser

Natural Healing for Women is written by two people with many years experience in natural medicine. It explains the different needs of our energy and repair systems and how to use the natural healing options now available. It is fully comprehensive and easy to use, and it includes:

The Repertory of Ailments: organised by the different body systems and areas of health, it covers psychological problems as well as physical ailments – from anxiety to acne and children's illnesses to cancer – and explains conventional methods of treatment and the benefits of alternative approaches.

The Materia Medica: an A to Z of alternative remedies and treatments, including homoeopathy, herbal and flower remedies and essential oils, with clear instructions on preparation and application.

Lifestyle: a unique guide to healing mind, body and spirit. It contains realistic guidelines for improving diet, exercise, sleep and relaxation techniques, complete with a cleansing programme and useful first aid kit.

For a natural approach to total well-being there is no better book.

The Audre Lorde Compendium
Essays, speeches and journals
Introduced by Alice Walker

When Audre Lorde died in 1992 the world mourned the passing of one of the giants of the feminist movement. Dedicated to activism through communication, she was described by Adrienne Rich as 'the Amazon warrior who also knows how to tell the tale of battle'.

This compendium collects together for the first time the essays, speeches and journals first published in *Sister Outsider*, *The Cancer Journals* and *A Burst of Light*. Including such classics as 'Uses of the erotic', 'The master's tools will never dismantle the master's house' and 'A Burst of Light: Living with Cancer', this collection shows the passion, humanity and towering courage of a woman always 'at the cutting edge of consciousness'.

'Lorde's works will be important to all those truly interested in growing up sensitive, intelligent and aware in the second half of the twentieth century.'
New York Times

'Audre Lorde's words of love and wisdom and courage give me strength.'
Alice Walker